Reflective Practice in Child and Adolescent Psychotherapy

Therapy referrals for a child or young person can be motivated for a number of reasons. The parents, carers or professionals responsible for their wellbeing might describe a sudden change in presentation, risk taking behaviour, such as self-harm or experimentation with drugs, alcohol or sex, or they might label the young person as over reacting, under reacting or attention seeking. Such behaviour prompts concern for their safety and confusion about why the child or young person is presenting the way they are. This book offers a thoughtful approach to making sense of such behaviour and encourages adults to 'reflect on' rather than 'react to' young peoples' outward presentations.

Based on the author's work with children, young people and families over two decades, this book shares reflections from the therapy room and illustrates how the therapist can try to make sense of mood, behaviour and presentations that previously made no sense. The content relies heavily on clinical experience as well as drawing on classical and contemporary psychotherapeutic literature.

So often adults find themselves reacting to observable behaviour in a judgmental or punitive way, rather than pausing to consider what the behaviour might be communicating. The author aims to model a thoughtful reflective approach to making sense of what might be going on for children and young people and this book will be of great interest to child and adolescent psychotherapists, related professionals and those with an interest in young persons' mental health.

Jeanine Connor is a child and adolescent psychotherapist, supervisor and trainer in private practice with a special interest in children, adolescents and looked after children. She is editor of BACP Children, Young People & Families and a regular contributor to BACP Therapy Today. Jeanine has previously worked in educational settings and in Child and Adolescent Mental Health Services (CAMHS).

'This powerful, concentrated book captures the essence of psycho-dynamic practice with children, young people and their families today. These kids bring unimaginable lives of indifference, betrayal, neglect and abuse, or sometimes just incomprehension, from those charged with their care. Jeanine Connor decries lazy labelling and eschews the fairy-tale ending; rather, she leaves threads so the reader – whether student, experienced practitioner or, indeed, parent – can explore, quarrel with and unravel her insightful interpretations and interventions. Alongside are helpful references to beacon texts from the literature. These stories celebrate the role of the therapist – listening, absorbing, containing, understanding and ultimately, we hope, freeing.'

Catherine Jackson, Editor,
BACP Therapy Today

'For any aspiring therapist working with children and young people, this book demonstrates how to be both firm and kind, how to combine clear theoretical thinking with human compassion and a flexibility of approach. This is an accessible, unpretentious book, distilling many years of wise practice with young clients. I recommend it to all therapists learning how best to work with the turbulence of adolescence.'

Nick Luxmoore, Psychotherapist,
Supervisor, Trainer and Author

Reflective Practice in Child and Adolescent Psychotherapy

Listening to Young People

Jeanine Connor

Routledge
Taylor & Francis Group

LONDON AND NEW YORK

First published 2020
by Routledge
2 Park Square, Milton Park, Abingdon, Oxon OX14 4RN

and by Routledge
52 Vanderbilt Avenue, New York, NY 10017

Routledge is an imprint of the Taylor & Francis Group, an informa business

© 2020 Jeanine Connor

British Library Cataloguing-in-Publication Data
A catalogue record for this book is available from the British
Library

Library of Congress Cataloging-in-Publication Data
A catalog record has been requested for this book

ISBN: 978-0-367-14939-0 (hbk)
ISBN: 978-0-367-14940-6 (pbk)
ISBN: 978-0-429-05402-0 (ebk)

Typeset in Times New Roman
by codeMantra

This book is dedicated to all the children, young people and families who have generously shared their stories with me. It is always a privilege to listen and to help them to make sense of it.

Contents

Disclaimer

This book is based on an amalgamation of therapeutic experiences with hundreds of children, young people, families and professionals over a period of more than two decades. No individual, family or organisation is recognisable by name or narrative.

Preface

I met a mother and son recently for an initial psychotherapy consultation. Twelve-year-old Aaron wasn't sure whether he wanted
therapy or how or if it could help him. He had a very good point;
how *could* he know how helpful it could be when he had no idea
what therapy was like and what would happen in the room. Aaron's
mother told me that she'd been concerned about her son for about
six months. He'd been getting into fights at school and had been
stealing money, mostly from her purse. The crunch point that led
to her seeking professional support – there is always a crunch point,
an answer to the 'why now?' question – was that Aaron was on
the brink of exclusion from school and had recently been caught
shoplifting in the local village Co-op. I wondered what his mother
thought the behaviour might be about, what sense she made of it.
She said it didn't make any sense at all; Aaron had always been such
a good boy and she felt he had everything that he needed. I noticed
that Aaron had lowered his head as his mother and I were talking
and I thought that he looked teary eyed. I asked him what sense *he*
made of the changes in his behaviour and he acknowledged that it
made no sense to him either. I told Aaron and his mother that my
work as a psychotherapist is about helping children, young people
and their families to make sense of things that don't make sense to
them. I shared that I already had some thoughts about what might
be going on for Aaron. He raised his head and looked at me curiously then said,

Therapy sounds like a good idea. Let's give it a try.

Readers might recognise my name as one that's been printed in
professional journals over the last decade or so. You might recall

my articles in which I've tried to make sense of shitty families, constipated systems, violent computer games and plenty of sex-related stuff that has been stimulated by my work as a psychotherapist working with children, young people and families. I often find myself reflecting on and making sense of things that are not usually spoken about, either in print or in person. I am someone with whom that which cannot usually be talked about *can*. Working with children and young people that is a really important point to make explicit from the start. They can – and they do – talk to me about a whole range of things that they have been struggling to find someone to talk about with. Psychotherapy is described as a 'talking therapy', which, in my experience on both sides of the 'couch', feels like a misnomer. I, like many other psychotherapists, do infinitely less talking than I do listening. So much so that I think 'listening therapy' would be a more fitting title for the work that I do. I have been listening to children, young people and their families in a professional capacity for over twenty years. My experience has taught me an immeasurable amount about what they think, feel and do regarding life, sex, death and everything in between. By young people I mean children and adolescents, which requires further clarification because meanings vary according to legal, cultural and biological definitions. The United Nations Convention on the Rights of a Child defines a child as someone below the age of eighteen years, a definition agreed by 192 of the 194 member countries. The Children Act (1989) also states that a person becomes a legal adult on their eighteenth birthday, and agrees that anyone under that age is legally a child. Children generally have fewer rights than adults, are deemed less able to make serious decisions and must legally be under the care of a parent or other responsible adult acting 'in loci parentis'. They do have responsibilities though. The age of criminal responsibility in England, Wales and Northern Ireland is ten while in Scotland it's eight. That's a confusing message – you're ten years away from adulthood, longer than your current lifetime, but you can be held responsible for committing a crime. There is a lot about being a young person that is confusing. There are also variations to the definition cross-culturally. For example in Singapore, a child is legally defined as someone under the age of fourteen (Children and Young Persons Act, 2008), while according to US Immigration Law (2000), a child refers to an unmarried person under the age of twenty-one. So, as with all vocabulary, we cannot assume that 'child' means the same thing to everyone, particularly if we are working cross-culturally.

Biologically, childhood denotes the stage of development from birth to puberty and in some definitions it includes the period pre-birth. The time spent in utero is becoming more widely recognised as significant in what follows afterwards for children and young people, and it continues to influence us into adulthood. When I am beginning a new sense-making journey with a child or young person I always start there: in utero. They can't tell me about it themselves, of course, but I always ask their parent or parents about the pregnancy and birth, questions such as who was around, how did it go, what were those first days, weeks and months like for your baby and you. I also ask about the parental relationship and the conception – was it planned or longed for, how did parents and siblings respond to the news? If the child or young person is adopted, fostered or in another care arrangement, I still ask questions about their conception, birth and early years. As well as providing useful context to what is going on in the here-and-now, this kind of exploration also illustrates the importance of the family around the child. The psychoanalyst Donald Winnicott said,

> There is no such thing as a baby... if you set out to describe a baby, you will find you are describing a baby and someone.
>
> (Winnicott, 1957)

What he meant by that was that a baby cannot exist in isolation and so too, the child or young person cannot - and should not - be considered in isolation either. If we have any hope of making sense of what is going on for the individual in therapy, we must also try to make sense of what is going on, or has gone on, with the family.

Many cultures perceive puberty as a transition from childhood to adulthood and mark this with a rite of passage. For example, Jewish boys celebrate their Bar Mitvah at age thirteen while Jewish girls celebrate Bat Mitzvah slightly earlier aged twelve. In Central and South America, fifteen-year-old girls celebrate Quinceanera, a ritual involving the renewal of vows made at their baptism in a Catholic mass that symbolises their commitment to family and faith. Inuit boys aged eleven or twelve traditionally go out hunting with their fathers to test their skills and acclimatise to the harsh arctic weather. For young people raised in the Amish tradition, their sixteenth birthday marks the beginning of Rumspringa. They are encouraged to enjoy unsupervised time away from their family experiencing the world beyond their culture for a period that can

last up to ten years! To me, this sounds like a most excellent idea –
ten years to explore and experiment with other people their age,
without parents or carers helicoptering over their shoulder. Those
Amish adolescents who choose to return to their community are
baptized as committed members of the Amish culture, marking the
end of Rumspringa. While some of these rituals and rites of passage might seem peculiar, they clearly denote, and in most cultures
celebrate, the transition between childhood and adulthood. In most
Western cultures, however, the transition tends to be more ambiguous and less celebrated. It is no surprise then that children and adolescents themselves, as well as those of us involved with providing
care and support, have a sense of ambiguity too.

Adolescence is the transitional stage between childhood and
adulthood that involves physical, social, intellectual, emotional
and psychological development. The term is derived from the Latin
adolescere, which means 'to grow up' – something adolescents are
often told to do by parents, carers and teachers. Wherever they
live and whatever social norms their lives are shaped by, there is
so much going on for adolescents. Their bodies are changing shape
and size. Their hormones are influencing their moods and behaviours. They are confronted with pressure from peers, parents,
teachers, media and social media to conform, perform and achieve.
And, not surprisingly, many children and young people struggle
with these internal and external pressures and find themselves in
need of support.

Reflective practice is the basis of my work as a child and adolescent
psychotherapist and it is a theme I emphasise in my auxiliary roles as
a supervisor, trainer and writer, as well as in consultations with parents, carers and other professionals. The term 'reflective practice' is
bandied around quite a bit and seems to mean something different to
different people. For me, reflective practice is about being thoughtful
and contemplative. It is about working collaboratively and in part-
nership with the child or young person and their family, directly or
indirectly, and it is about listening, really listening, to what they have
to say. So often, children and young people find themselves in situations where they do not feel listened to and where they feel that their
voices are not being heard. Maybe that is why some of them shout
so loudly and why others stop bothering to say anything compre-
hensible at all and resort to grunts. I have lost count of the number
of young people who have said to me, 'no-one ever listens' and it can
feel peculiar to them when someone finally does.

When I listen to young people in psychotherapy I am not just listening to what they say. I am also listening to the tone, the manner, the words and vocabulary, their use of language, sarcasm and swearing – yes, swearing is totally permitted in my therapy room! As I listen, I notice themes and nuances, contemplate them and reflect them back so I can think about them together with the child or young person in the room and start to make sense of what they might mean. I am also 'listening' to what is not said; the things that children and young people are unable or unwilling to verbalise, and I reflect on that too. So often, adults find themselves in a position of 'reacting to' rather than 'reflecting with' children and young people. This is not a criticism; I know it can be an instinctive response to a young person who is reacting too. I am thinking here in particular about the acting-out child, the argumentative pre-teen or the boundary-testing adolescent. It is common to react to these kinds of reactive behaviours in a judgmental (at best) or punitive (at worst) way, rather than pausing to make sense of it and considering what the young person's words or behaviour might be trying to communicate. But this is seldom helpful and it sets up a pattern of relationships where everyone reacts, no one listens, nothing makes sense and nothing changes. The aim of sharing my experiences as a child and adolescent psychotherapist in this book is to encourage adults to listen, reflect and make sense of rather than react to children and young people's communications. By doing so, we are all much better equipped to get alongside them, think with them, work with them collaboratively and help them to make sense of things. This models a thoughtful, healthy way of relating to each other and leads to improvements in children and young peoples' emotional and psychological health. When they feel listened to, children and young people are enabled to learn, develop and relate with other people more healthily because everything starts to make better sense.

As a child and adolescent psychotherapist, my role is to help children and young people to acknowledge, reflect upon and make sense of what is going on, or what has gone on, in their lives. My model of working is psychodynamic in orientation, which means that I believe that the unconscious greatly influences what we say and do. The unconscious part of the mind contains relics of past experiences, which continue to influence us in the present, and can manifest in word, thought, behaviour, play, drawings, dreams and jokes. The motivation for much of what happens in sessions (and in life per se) is beyond conscious awareness. For those people without a psychodynamic training this can be a difficult concept to understand. For me, it is about the distinction between the content of the session; what is said and done – and the process; the feelings that occur within and between us. In psychotherapy sessions with children and young people I notice recurrent themes, mannerisms, feeling responses (mine and theirs) slips of the tongue (ditto) and note my observations about what might be happening both consciously and unconsciously. I also help children and young people to make links between past and present feelings and experiences and to become more aware of the unconscious processes at play. This enables a better understanding of what might be going on for them so that it makes sense and so that change can happen. After all, most people come into therapy because they want something to change. Becoming aware of unconscious processes, which can manifest in repetitive patterns of unhelpful or unhealthy behaviour or recurrent issues, can enable children and young people to better manage their emotions and experiences, make safer choices, have healthier relationships, achieve better mental health and live happier, more rewarding lives. As one child said to me,

> I don't really understand how therapy works, but it feels like magic.

I am inclined to agree.

In order to help children and young people to engage in therapy and explore the contents of their conscious and unconscious minds I have a variety of resources available to them, as well as talking and listening. Contrary to the traditional idea about psychodynamic psychotherapy, my room is much more than a blank, impersonal space. I have comfortable furniture and the walls are decorated with colour and pictures. Some of the resources, such as books and art materials, are on display and easily accessible. Others, such as clay, games and musical instruments, are housed in cupboards waiting to be discovered. The feeling that I hope to portray is one of a warm, welcoming and containing space and most of the children and young people I work with sense that as soon as they arrive. Many will comment on the room and most appreciate the effort I have made with them in mind. Sometimes though it can be difficult for them to understand why I would bother. One adolescent I worked with asked me,

> Why would you have a nice room like this for people like me?

His question was communicating his sense of worthlessness, which was an enduring theme of therapy for him.

Very many books have been written about child and adolescent psychotherapy. Some offer how-to models of working therapeutically, and some include self-help and parenting strategies. Others provide theoretical perspectives, research findings or focus on treating specific disorders. Those books certainly have their worth and there are many of them on my own bookshelves. But this book is different. This book is an amalgamation of my real world experiences of helping children and young people to make sense of their real world issues such as loss, self-harm, online and offline relationships, friendships, death and sex. I explore these themes, and others, with reference to my work and I model ways to listen, reflect and make sense of, rather than react to what is presented. I refer to individual children and young people by name but these are unrecognisable amalgamations containing fragments of many different individuals in order to protect the confidentiality of the hundreds of families I have met through my work. While I have divided the book into chapters, you will notice common themes, threads and overlaps within and between them. Children and young people cannot and should not be put into boxes and, similarly, their behaviour does not fit neatly into any particular box either. That is what makes them so fascinating and complex and challenging. So, you will notice that I mention one theme in a chapter about another, while sex and relationships seem to crop up everywhere, just as they do in the real world.

Within each chapter, I share insights into what happens in psychotherapy with children, young people and their families including how I think with and about them, how I manage dilemmas and how I formulate my responses. I hope you will learn from this model of relating to children and young people and find it helpful in your own relationships with them. That said, this book is not intended to be a how-to manual. My therapeutic orientation is non-directional and I write with the same intent. I illustrate throughout the chapters how I listen, think, reflect and make sense with children and young people in therapy and I encourage you, the reader, to 'listen' to what I have to say, and then think, reflect and make sense of it in your own way. I have a quote in my therapy room that is precariously assigned to Buddha. Children and young people are intrigued when I refer to it as a reminder that I am not the expert about their lives; they are. The take away message that I hope to portray is that while I will certainly share my thoughts and ideas with them, they should only take from that what makes sense for them. I think it is also a useful quote to have in mind as you read this (and any other) book and consider what 'fits' with your own sensibilities,

> Believe nothing, no matter where you read it, or who said it, no matter if I have said it, unless it agrees with your own reason and your own common sense.

References

Children Act (1989) UK Parliament, London.
Children and Young Persons Act (2008) UK Parliament, London.
United Nations Convention on the Rights of a Child (1992) UNICEF, London.
US Immigration Law (2000) US Department of Justice, Washington, DC.
Winnicott, D. W. (1957) *The Child and the Outside World: Studies in Developing Relationships*, Tavistock, London.

Chapter 1

Psychotherapy with children, young people and families

Psychotherapy with children and young people is different to psychotherapy with adults. It requires a different set of skills and a different kind of patience and perseverance. It is infinitely more complex than working with adults because a child is always part of a family system in some shape or form that will be involved in the therapeutic work both directly and indirectly. The child and I will welcome some involvement from the family, while other involvement can feel intrusive or sabotaging. Sometimes I work with a parent and child together; other times just a parent or parents to support them to think about their child's difficulties. When I offer individual work to a child or young person I always include the parents or carers at the beginning and the end and at review points throughout the therapeutic intervention. It is important for parents and carers to feel as if they are included in the wok; they are responsible for their child's safety, including emotional safety, and they too might be struggling to make sense of what is going on for their child. I am not a substitute parent, I am a psychotherapist and we have different yet complementary roles. It is important to acknowledge that to parents and carers from the start; some of whom think it is my job to 'fix' their child and then hand them back without taking any responsibility themselves. Others feel pushed out by this new adult in their child's life who their child is opening up to in ways they can only dream of. These are extreme ends of the parental spectrum, of course, and most parents fall somewhere in between. They want to make sense of their child's behaviour, thoughts and feelings, and they want to have a better relationship with them, but they are struggling to know how to achieve that. The other thing that is important to note is that psychotherapy changes people and this has a ripple effect on the people around the person in therapy: the people in their family system. I sometimes use the analogy of a machine made up of cogs, a bit like the inside of a clock, to describe a family system. If one of those cogs – the child in therapy – changes shape, it might not fit with the other cogs the way it once did and they too will have to adjust their shape to make sure the machine can still function effectively. Just as cogs in a machine, people in families impact every other component in their system.

A lot of my work is with children who no longer live with their birth family because they are in foster or residential care. Looked after children often have multiple families that get 'brought' to therapy one way or another – in reality, in fantasy, in thought, in play or in the transference relationship. Their system is made up of previous and current carers as well as previous and current social care professionals. All of these adults will have had an impact on the young person and he or she on them. A lot of looked after children get moved around an awful lot between family systems and so they are constantly being expected to change shape in order to fit in with a differently shaped machine. Often this is too difficult and they get moved again. Often they don't know how to fit in with a new family because they don't know what shape they are expected to fit into. Often, by the time I meet them in therapy, they are confused about their own identity, shut off emotionally and highly defended against forming another relationship with another adult, not knowing what they expect from them either.

Jay

So what is psychotherapy with children and young people actually like? Those I work with often use metaphor to describe their experiences of psychotherapy. Some mention the 'wounds' they have suffered, and liken the therapeutic process to 'picking at' or 'uncovering' something difficult. This sounds painful, and of course therapy often is. Some children and young people try to protect their emotional wounds with a psychological sticking plaster. This is an attempt to cover up the hurt but we both know it is still there, just beneath the surface. As ten-year-old Jay told me in an initial session,

> If I take the plaster off now, it will just bleed and the badness will fester away inside me.

I think this was his way of telling me he wasn't ready to show me his wounds yet, which I respected, and that he wasn't sure if he was ready or able to heal, or whether therapy would be able to help him. It is important to acknowledge the client's uncertainty about therapy and mine too because I can never be sure whether a young person will find therapy helpful, no matter how much I want that to be true. Jay was also alerting me to the 'badness' he felt he had inside of him that was festering away and preventing him from healing. There was also a warning that if the plaster was removed too soon he would bleed; alerting me to the fact that it could get messy and that he couldn't be sure whether either of us could handle that just yet. What Jay bravely shared with me in that initial meeting was that his wounds were real, hurting and disgusting. I listened to his communication and I respected it. Jay and I worked together for twelve months exploring and making sense of, mostly through play and metaphor, his early experience of sexual abuse.

Jack

Another boy of the same age, Jack, arrived at his first session and showed me all the cuts and bruises on his legs that he had sustained through playing football. This became a ritual at the start of every session as he became increasingly committed in his determination to up the bruise count each week. Sometimes I struggled to see the tiniest of abrasions that Jack insisted were there. One week he asked if I had any plasters. I did, in a small first aid kit I keep on hand. He took out a strip and spent the session locating his bruises and sticking plasters over them. By the end of the session he had used up the whole pack! The next week, having replaced my stock of plasters, we went through the same ritual of locating and counting cuts and bruises on Jack's legs. By about the fifth session I was invited to put the plasters on Jack's legs instead of him doing it for himself. When a pattern of behaviour is repeated in therapy it is important to stay with it and observe. When it changes, however subtly, it marks a psychological shift. What happened in the first weeks of Jack's therapy felt like a deeply symbolic process. I was invited by Jack to acknowledge his wounds. Some were clear to see but others were barely visible although he insisted they were there. I listened to his communication and acknowledged that it felt important to him for me to see his injuries. This is symbolic of what can often happen in therapy. A young person is referred with a presenting issue – the wound that is clear to see – yet over time, other wounds show up that were less apparent or which the young person had kept hidden. With Jack, I made comments like,

> I can see some of these bruises really clearly, but others are harder for me to see.

This was true but non-shaming. I wasn't saying the other bruises weren't there, just that I struggled to see them. I wondered about the symbolic communication of witnessing Jack covering up his wounds with plasters. Perhaps he was saying,

> You can't help me, I have to do this for myself.

Or perhaps he was telling me,

> I'm keeping some of this hidden from you for now.

When the plasters ran out, I experienced a strong sense that my meagre resources might be an insufficient match for Jack's multiple layers of pain. It is not uncommon for me to wonder – and sometimes worry – about whether I will be able to help a child or young person when I meet them for the first time. But with Jack I felt this more strongly which suggests I was experiencing a projection of his own fears and anxieties about how helpful therapy could be. He was pleasantly surprised when I replenished the stocks in readiness for his next session and I think he understood my response (symbolically) as a communication that it was ok to take what he needed from me and that he wouldn't use me up. When finally I was invited by Jack to share in the process of providing first-aid, it felt like the perfect metaphor for Jack's readiness to begin therapy – which is always a collaborative process of making sense and of healing.

Other children and young people arrive for their first session protected, not by a metaphorical sticking plaster, but by much strong psychological defences that have served to protect them from emotional and sometimes physical pain. They might liken these defences to shields or armour or 'one million metre high walls', which was one young person's, not so subtle, way of warning me to keep out. It is important to acknowledge these communications and respect young people's defences. Stealing away their shield or asking them to remove their armour would leave them vulnerable, while taking a metaphorical sledgehammer to the walls they have spent years erecting could replicate earlier psychological damage and remove any hope of building a therapeutic relationship. If the time is right for a child or young person to start treatment, and only they can know this, I respect the defences that have served them well enough for long enough. I position myself alongside them as they start to slowly remove the plaster or take down the walls, brick by brick and reveal the wounds beneath in their own time. For some children and young people, like Jack, this can take weeks and for others it takes months or even years. According to the child or young person's own agenda of time, we examine the wounds as and when they are ready and we make the therapeutic journey together.

I remember being encouraged as a trainee therapist to have faith in the therapeutic process. I had no trouble comprehending the theory but this thing my tutors called the 'process' was an enigma. I think now that it is about disentangling the *content* of therapy from the *thinking-about* therapy. Initially, most of the processing happens outside of the consulting room in private reflection and/ or in supervision, but with increased clinical experience, the doing and the thinking-about become reconciled. For me, the process has a unique identity that is linked to, yet also distinct from, the content. I often find myself thinking about this with parents and carers of the children and young people I work with and it can be a difficult concept to explain and understand. Not surprisingly, the adults around the client want to know what happens in therapy and, more importantly, whether it is working. It can be difficult for them to comprehend what isn't tangible and to have faith in a process they aren't privy too. Most children and young people I work with seem to 'get' the therapeutic process instinctively. They can sense it, even though most of them would struggle, as I sometimes do, to explain its 'magical' quality. But there are some children and young people whose conscious or unconscious intention is to attack the process, such as the child who wants *me* to set the agenda, or the concrete-thinker who draws me into philosophical debate or logical argument in lieu of emotional connection. Or the young people who fill the session with talking and over-explaining and over-detailed accounts of he-said/she-said. In sessions such as these I find it hard to concentrate on what is being said, frightened I might mishear or misremember something when I write up my notes later. But then I remind myself that the verbatim account of what happened – or didn't happen, who am I to say? – is not what's important. What is important is how the session *feels*, what sense I make of it, or not. It is more important to notice the process of what's going on than get caught up in trying and failing to listen to the content, which is serving as a defence. Children and young people who fill the session up are keeping the emotional parts of themselves shut-off and trying to keep the thinking part of me shut-out. This is part of the process too, of course. Although it can be difficult to sit with, that is what I am being invited to do in these sessions. When I feel as if I'm being drawn into, or pushed away from something, I try to keep the thinking-part of myself alive and provide a commentary to the here-and-now. I might say something like,

> It seems like it's easier for us to think together today rather than feel.

Or,

> I'm getting a sense that you don't want me to think very much today.

That way I'm reflecting on the process, even though the young person is trying their best to sabotage it. This is often unconscious on their part, and comes as a consequence of well-practiced strategies that serve to protect them from painful emotions. As with other defences, I respect them but I do not ignore them. I say what I notice but I don't force a young person to go where they are not yet ready to go. It is their process, not mine.

There are other children and young people for whom the avoidance of the process is more blatant. The boy who yelled at me,

> Why do you have to analyse everything I say?

And the adolescent who screamed,

> There is no such thing as the fucking unconscious!

right in my face.

These young people were focussing on the content of the session and finding it difficult to contemplate the process. Perhaps that would have been too unbearable.

Priya

The antithesis of the child or young person who attacks the process with filling up the content is the one who creates an empty void. I understand this as an unconscious replication of the psychological empty void they carry internally. I remember an early adolescent client, Priya, who I worked with many years ago for several months. She attended every session and mostly sat in silence while I mostly sat in silence too. I didn't know what to do. I didn't know if therapy was helping her or whether I should continue seeing her. I reduced her sessions from weekly to fortnightly because I thought the frequency might feel too intimate and that it could be affecting her capacity to engage. I thought about ending therapy altogether because, well if I am honest, I didn't find it very satisfying. Every session left me feeling drained and often with a headache. It felt pointless. We weren't talking or doing anything and there is only so much silence I can listen to. I felt like I wasn't good enough. When I pushed aside the content and reflected instead on the process, I was able to understand it as a mirroring of Priya's experiences. Only then was I able to sense – and make sense of – what was going on.

Priya was a looked after child who had experienced multiple placements and been excluded from school. Her sixth social worker had resigned and not yet been replaced. She had sporadic contact with her parents who were separated and each had new partners and new children; Priya's half siblings who seemingly took priority over her in their parent's lives and minds. I felt an immense sadness in relation to Priya's repeated experience of rejection and abandonment. I thought her sense of being un-wantable must be overwhelming and her projections so powerful that I hadn't wanted her and had considered abandoning her too. It is remarkable how the therapeutic relationship mirrored Priya's other relationships where contact had been reduced or terminated and where new siblings had replaced her. I had also considered getting rid of my unsatisfying client in order to make space for a new, potentially more rewarding one. But I contained Priya's projections week after week, which demonstrated to her my willingness to bear them. I had felt useless, hopeless and deskilled, just as she did, but I had endured those feelings alongside her. At other times I had felt punishing and hating but I had resisted the temptation to punish Priya by rejecting her. Much of the communication between Priya and me was unconscious and non-verbal, and most of what happened was in the rich therapeutic process rather than the empty-feeling content of the sessions. Priya must have sensed that too – why else would she have kept coming back? My feeling was that she experienced something nurturing in our therapeutic relationship. There was no agenda and no rules about right or wrong, she could just 'be' and perhaps, most powerfully of all, experience another person just being with her too. She had not said very much but I had still listened and made sense of her internal world. How valuable the therapeutic space must have been for Priya, a girl who lacked any consistent, dependable, safe spaces, and what a wonderful thing to be able to provide for her.

Trudy

My work with Priya mostly took place in the transference relationship at an unconscious level. There is always an unconscious element to communication, even when a young person communicates with words, as was the case with fourteen-year-old Trudy. If I'm totally honest, I experienced the adolescent as drab, untidy and a bit of a mess. I am not saying this disrespectfully, it is important to acknowledge our first impressions of clients because they contain an important communication. This can feel uncomfortable, which might also be saying something about the client's uncomfortable feelings too. When I ask new supervisees or inexperienced therapists to tell me about their clients' appearance they can often feel awkward and say something vague for fear of sounding judgemental, rude or stereotyping. In the real world we are taught from a young age that it is unacceptable to say or even think anything that could be perceived as negative about someone's appearance and this is a hard habit to break. But in the therapeutic space *all* our observations are grist for the mill and most psychotherapists come to realise the value of this through training, clinical experience and containing supervision. I am mindful to own – and encourage supervisees to own – my/their perceptions of a client's appearance rather than state those perceptions as fact, and it is interesting to notice any discrepancies.

I once worked with a young woman, Jacintha, in an educational setting, whom I perceived as incredibly attractive. In my mind she was glamorously dressed with fabulously styled hair and immaculate make up and nails. One week my supervisor noticed Jacintha walking away from my therapy room as she was arriving for our meeting. I told her, 'that's her, the beautiful one'. My supervisor said she would never have guessed and that, to her, the young woman looked decidedly ordinary, like countless other young women on campus. The important thing, the thing of therapeutic significance, was not what Jacintha actually looked like, but how I interpreted her appearance and presentation in the context of our therapeutic relationship – what Bion might have called 'the Jacintha in my mind' (Casement, 1985). As I unpicked this idea in supervision, I came to realise that I had idealised my client, who had also idealised me, and that we had got caught up in the positive transference. As I began to disentangle myself, the 'beautiful one' did indeed become more ordinary looking (to me), allowing space for the more ordinary and the less beautiful parts of herself to become known about in therapy.

Anyway, back to Trudy. Perhaps what I was picking up from her in my initial interpretations of her appearance was that she felt a bit of a mess herself. She lived with her maternal grandparents who loved her unconditionally and did their best to take care of her. But despite the new clothes and the pretty accessories, she just didn't present in the same way as the other girls her age. It wasn't that appearance didn't matter to Trudy because every week she complimented me on mine with comments such as,

You look nice today – I like your hair – Are those new shoes?

She was always polite and smiley and we explored her desire to be liked. In the real world, outside of therapy, Trudy had difficult relationships with her peers. When I first met her she presented a narrative of herself as well-liked and popular, with lots of girlfriends and her pick of potential boyfriends. It didn't ring true. I meet lots of young people of Trudy's age and I could not imagine many of them wanting to hang out with her based on my first impressions. Trudy was incredibly observant and we explored the ways her vigilance linked to her earlier experiences. She knew that I knew about the neglect she had experienced as a younger child. Her mother, who was not much older when she had Trudy than Trudy was when I met her, had been unable to meet her daughter's basic needs. As a consequence, Trudy was often left unkempt and unfed. She knew that I knew this, but she found it difficult to acknowledge, believing that to do so would be disrespectful towards her mother, whom she desperately loved and harboured a desire to go back and live with. But of course Trudy did share something of her experience with me in the way that she presented herself. Therapy is never about apportioning blame, but for young people like Trudy in can feel like that and so it is important to tread carefully. I might say something like,

> Your mum did the best that she could

because usually mums do. I honestly do not believe that anyone sets out to intentionally be a bad mother, or even one that is less than good enough, but sometimes that happens. I think that Trudy's compliments spoke something about our relationship that by focusing solely on her story I could have missed. What she was communicating was that she noticed I bothered to tidy up my hair and think about my clothes before I met with her, which in turn, demonstrated that I thought she was worth the effort. Her comments could therefore be interpreted as gratitude – 'thanks for caring enough to bother'. I knew from her narrative that not everyone paid her this level of respect. She mentioned the Saturday she met her mum for breakfast. Her mother was described as scruffily dressed in tracksuit and trainers but had a dress and sandals in her bag to change into before she went shopping with a friend in the afternoon. She mentioned a teacher who showed her the jacket she had purchased at lunchtime but quipped that it was much too nice to wear to school. Other peoples' appearances were important to Trudy. Her compliments about mine communicated something about what it symbolised for her about our relationship. So when she complimented me on how I looked it wasn't really about *me*, it was about *us*. Her unconscious communication was something like,

> I've noticed you care about me and I'm grateful

because we both knew that not everyone did.

The relationship

Therapy fulfils a primitive human need to be connected to someone who is connected to us. It does other things as well but the therapeutic relationship is the fundamental thing. All the research agrees that the relationship is what matters most, not the model of therapy, the theoretical discipline or the duration. The relationship between therapist and client has theoretical comparisons to that between infant and mother, no matter what the gender of the individuals involved. The infant needs food, warmth and shelter if it is to survive, but what it needs most of all is love. As Sue Gerhardt says in her excellent book – 'love matters' (2004). The child or young person in therapy also needs to feel loved by their therapist. Some people find that controversial but I do not understand why. It is not sexual love I am describing but parental love and no one should have a problem with that. As a therapist, I am often on the receiving end of loving projections from clients, particularly those children and young people, like Trudy, who crave a loving parental relationship. I reciprocate by loving them back, in the maternal, nurturing sense, because love matters; it enables children to thrive and to survive. Sometimes people ask me how I can do what I do without getting emotionally involved with or attached to the children and young people I work with. The truth is I cannot and I do not want to. If I did not feel an emotional connection towards my clients they would not feel held or cared about by me. They would sense that I was 'just doing a job' and they would 'just do a job' too. They would turn up and they might engage at a superficial level but we would not be able to form a relationship. I hear from children and young people about their previous experiences with professionals and professional carers, sometimes with biological and step-parents who 'go through the motions' of providing the basics – food, shelter, resources – but they don't feel loved by them and they don't feel known or understood. In order to know and understand a child or young person we need to develop the capacity to be engaged by them.

The psychotherapist Donald Winnicott coined the phrase 'maternal preoccupation' (1986) initially to denote the period of early infancy. He stated that the new mother must be in tune with her baby psychologically and biologically in order to make sense of and respond to their needs. The attuned mother does not have to be preoccupied with their baby every second of every day, because the baby also needs to learn how to manage separation, frustration and longing. Winnicott talked about the 'good enough' mother and the 'good enough' experience of the infant. If the baby does not experience 'good enough' mothering it is unable to develop a sense of itself as a separate being that feels loved and has its needs met. Many of the children and young people who are referred to therapy have not had a good enough experience of maternal preoccupation. But therapy can provide this experience for them as well as the opportunity for reparation. The therapist is a different kind of mother – male or female – who can be totally preoccupied with their 'infant' client, no matter what their age. Some children and young people, adolescents in particular, can find this uncomfortable if their earliest experience of being mothered was less than good-enough. While it is the norm for them to have hundreds if not thousands of online 'friends' the idea of being connected with someone whose primary concern is them for a whole therapeutic hour can feel intimidating and exposing and cringe-making. That is often why they need to leave the room countless times to go to the bathroom, or they arrive late or leave early; it's just *too* intimate. But the experience of maternal preoccupation can also feel exquisite. That sense of feeling connected, once they are attuned to it, can be wonderful. It feels nice to be with someone who wants to be with you. We experience things together, we review past experiences and we look forward to times we will spend together in the future. As therapists we are attuned to the here-and-now of our sessions with clients, the relationship in time between the two people in the room.

Zak

The power of the relationship brings to mind my work with eight-year-old Zak. The school's family liaison officer described him to me as unteachable, unreachable and uncommunicative. Zak's mother 'forgot' to bring him to his first session and I sat in my therapy room thinking about him in his absence. When I did eventually meet Zak I was able to state honestly that I had held him in mind. Not surprisingly, he struggled to comprehend this or to communicate his thoughts and feelings. Nevertheless, Zak attended ten therapy sessions where he experienced a different kind of parent/child relationship and something shifted. He began spending time with his family instead of in his room. He invited a friend home for the first time in eight years and his academic performance improved dramatically. I was informed that therapy had done its magic! I think the 'magic' that Zak responded to was 'maternal preoccupation', which can feel enchanting indeed.

I've referred to a number of first sessions in this chapter and will continue to do so throughout this book. First sessions, like any first meeting, contain a wealth of information about how the relationship is likely to pan out. Everything about them is fascinating – how they get set up and by whom. Who attends and who doesn't. Whether they turn up on time, stay for the duration, leave early or try to overstay the boundary of their session time. Who sits where and what they say or don't say. And of course what is most fascinating of all is how the first session *feels*, before, during and after the fifty-minute slot. First meetings with anyone, a potential partner, employer, or client can feel anxiety provoking, nerve-wracking and exciting. The sense I make of a first session and what I am left with afterwards is crucial to note. What gets set up often sets up the themes for the therapy, and this usually starts with how first sessions are set up themselves.

Sarah

Sarah contacted me about her eleven-year-old daughter, Millie, via my online referral form. In the space where it asked how she had heard about me she wrote,

A local lady recommended you

which was both ambiguous and intriguing. I wondered why she did not want to say who the local lady was. I recognized that something about Sarah's vagueness suggested that she wanted to keep parts of herself and her external world away from me. I offered a first appointment for mother, daughter and me, as is my usual practice for initial consultations, but Sarah wanted to meet me alone. She said there were things she wanted to talk about to do with Millie that she did not want to say in front of her daughter. This was further suggestion of Sarah's need to keep things separate, although I did wonder why she would want to keep Millie separate from Millie's own therapy and potential therapist. Perhaps she wanted me to herself? I wondered too what Sarah needed to keep split-off psychologically and I acknowledged the anxiety she had displayed in her communication with me so far. Prior to our first appointment, Sarah asked to speak to me on the telephone. She told me she had read the therapeutic contract on my website and wanted to 'get a few things straight'. Mostly what had caught her attention was the part about confidentiality. She wanted a guarantee that I would let her know what Millie talked to me about in her individual sessions. I told her that I could not offer such reassurance because therapy is private, even from parents. Sarah really struggled with this, telling me that she was Millie's mother and therefore had every right to know what her daughter talked about. Sarah seemed so filled with anxiety that I had a sense of it spilling out down the telephone.

I did my best to assuage this by assuring her that, if I were to work with her daughter, she would be invited to regular reviews where we could think together about how therapy was going and any themes and patterns, but that what Millie chose to share, or not share, with her mother about the content of therapy was up to her. I had not even met Millie yet, let alone agreed to work with her, and it already felt as if her mother was sabotaging her therapy. I reminded myself that it was Sarah who had initially made contact with me and that this push/pull way of relating probably expressed both her ambivalence about therapy, as well as something about her other relationships. The telephone call with Sarah left me feeling exhausted and I approached our initial face-to-face meeting with a sense of dread.

Sarah arrived alone and precisely on time. She was a compact, buttoned-up woman who spoke in a clipped, efficient way as she recounted her life story. I had not asked for this, I had thought we were meeting to talk about Millie. She told me she had been let down by countless 'people like you' and that she had very low expectations about therapy. I remember thinking, 'I'll show you', but what I was *feeling*, despite being faced with this formidable, highly defended, verbally attacking woman in the room, was that I really wanted to help her to have a happier and more fulfilling life. And against the odds I did. I offered to work with Sarah and to refer her daughter to a colleague, which was agreed. We worked together for a year and she always arrived on time and never missed a session. Ours was an intense relationship but we survived it, learnt to love each other and gradually she thrived. When the day came to end, Sarah thanked me for bearing her and I thanked her in return for letting me in.

Marley

Thinking about what gets set up in first sessions brings to mind Marley, an outwardly confident eighteen-year-old full of strut and swagger. He was referred for help with emotional dysregulation and difficulty in relationships. Marley announced his arrival at our first session by hammering so loudly on the door I thought he might punch a hole through it. He was tall, broad and solid looking; physically attractive and conveying the impression that he knew it. Once inside, Marley relaxed into the couch, not waiting to be invited, and began chatting almost immediately. He seemed to take up a lot of space – both on the furniture and in the room – giving me a real sense of his large presence. He talked about his college course, his family, friends and girlfriends – there were plenty of those. I found him engaging and was delighted that he seemed comfortable enough to engage with me so openly and so quickly. The session flashed by and all too soon it was time to end. Marley stood up, shook my hand enthusiastically and swaggered off. I had found him intriguing and was really looking forward to us working together. The following week I waited for Marley and as the minutes ticked by the realization struck me that he wasn't coming. My initial feeling was one of disappointment, quickly followed by a sense that his disengagement was inevitable. I tried unsuccessfully to contact him. I left both a voice message and a text to say that I had kept him in mind and invited him to get in touch if he wanted to make another appointment. He didn't reply. Of course he didn't! On reflection, it seemed as if Marley had attempted to seduce me during our first (and only) meeting, with pseudo charm and faux intimacy and in a way it worked. I think that's how he operated; by using his physicality, masculinity and bravado to draw people in, only to immediately pull away, or push *them* away in order to avoid emotional intimacy. I should have known this was going to happen; he was emotionally dysregulated and had difficulty in relationships – yet I'd been beguiled. Our therapeutic relationship, like many of Marley's relationships, had no immediate future; he simply wasn't ready to commit. What gets played out in the therapy room so often mimics what has gone before, particularly in terms of the relationship.

Amber

Amber was in her mid-teens and, like Marley, she seemed to engage enthusiastically during our first session. She had many questions about me to do with my age, how long I'd been a therapist, my marital and parental status as well as whether or not I smoked or liked 'grime' – she was referring to music rather than muck. Her questions didn't feel interrogating, they felt fair enough, and I was delighted that she had the confidence to be so openly curious. Amber told me about her previous counsellors, whom she referred to as Bellend 1 and Bellend 2. She said that Bellend 1 always made her a cup of tea and provided biscuits, while Bellend 2 let her smoke when they walked Bellend 2's dog together. I worried that I'd already been placed in the role of Bellend 3 and that I would be judged harshly for my therapeutic boundaries against these real or imagined predecessors who had apparently given Amber so much. The following session Amber arrived a few minutes late and with much less enthusiasm. She wanted to know if I had something for her to eat and drink. I said I didn't and reminded her that we don't eat or drink in the therapy room. When I wondered how she had felt after the first session and about coming back for a second, she responded monosyllabically. Not long afterwards she fell asleep, a state she occupied for the remainder of the session. During the silence I reflected on our first meeting and realized that Amber hadn't told me anything about herself at all. Instead she'd employed a sophisticated form of defence that I had mistaken as engagement. Her catatonic state was less subtle and her communication in session two was loud and clear, despite her slumber. Amber was testing out ways to control what happened in therapy as well as ways to monitor how intimate we could be together. She was also testing my boundaries and I understood that despite her banging on them furiously she needed for me to keep them in place if we were to have any chance of developing a containing therapeutic relationship.

Kyle

It is worth making reference to how I manage requests from the children and young people I work with (and their parents or carers) for personal information about me. I know that different counsellors and psychotherapists have different rules about personal disclosure that are informed by professional discipline and individual inclination. Very few, especially those of us working with children and young people, occupy the traditionally psychoanalytic 'blank slate' position, and not many are willing to share everything they are asked to. I think we each have to find a position that feels comfortable enough in relation to each unique client situation. What I am most willing to share is what we think of nowadays as public domain information: anything that is available via a search engine to anyone who can spell my name. But to simply provide facts and figures type stuff to clients such as Amber without facilitating exploration is to miss a trick. I would argue that the questions themselves are always more revealing than the answers, or lack of answers, that we might provide. When I am asked about my own life (or not) during a therapy session it always tells me something about my client. One young man, Kyle, was particularly interrogational in his first session, wanting to know all about my childhood, my parents and siblings and whether I had been abused. Kyle had spent ten years in the care system with a not unrealistic belief that decisions were made for and about him rather than with his consent. He had been physically abused as a child and raped during early adolescence. He had suffered a lifetime of intrusion so it made sense that his questioning would feel intrusive as he projected his experiences onto me. Kyle told me it wasn't fair that I wanted to know all about him while he knew nothing at all about me. When I commented that his therapy was supposed to be about him not me he wasn't satisfied. In fact he was really unsatisfied and I knew he would not come back after the first session if I didn't give a little. So I attempted to negotiate. I said it made good sense for him to work out if he thought I could help him and in order to do that he needed to know about me. He visibly relaxed but held onto a healthy dose of scepticism, wanting to know why I was a psychotherapist 'dealing with other people's shit'. The real question, implicit in this remark, was whether I could deal with *his* shit. I let him know that this is what I thought he was wondering about and he smiled a little – probably because not only I had used the word 'shit' but also, I think, because I had bothered to make sense of what was implicit in his question.

One of the most important things I can offer to children and young people is empathy, both with their own experiences and with their curiosity about mine. So I am always willing to explore why it matters to them if my parents are alive or whether or not they abused me – and how my reality might relate to theirs. And I am equally willing to reflect on questions about whether I have taken drugs or smoked or been drunk – and how my reality might relate to theirs. I do not usually share anything that my clients could not find out for themselves and that becomes more bearable as they learn to understand that the sessions are about them. Gradually they see that my unwillingness to talk about me is not about withholding but the opposite; it is about holding the therapeutic boundaries and offering containment. I realised that Amber had finally understood this when in a much later session she said to me,

> I knew everything about my other counsellor; she had no boundaries!

It is important that counsellors and therapists, as well as parents and carers, recognise and hold the boundary between what is ours and what belongs to the child. That is one of the reasons why individual psychotherapy is so important for therapists in training prior to them offering therapy to clients, particularly, I think, if they are working or planning to work with children and young people. This client group stirs up all sorts of feelings in therapists about their own experiences of being mothered, whether that was good enough or not, and of being in relationships with their own children. It is vital to make sense of our own experiences and feelings about our experiences and to hold a boundary around them. Only then are we able to really be attuned to and have the capacity to hold the children and young people we work with. For me, the job of therapy is to make sense of things for the child or young person. This process is akin to Wilfred Bion's concept of 'maternal reverie' (1967). He described this as the mother's capacity to sense what is going on inside her baby and then make sense of it. We are better able to do this if we are aware of and have made sense of what is going on inside ourselves. Like the pre-verbal infant, the child or young person in therapy might not recognise what is going on for them, or they might recognise it but not have the words to describe it or the capacity to process it. I see it as my role to first of all sense what is going on inside the child or young person and then make sense of it with them in the space between us. It is always a privilege to be invited in to witness the internal world of a child or young person and to help them make sense of it. Not from a position of authority, but from alongside. Therapy is a creative process akin to playing together. As Winnicott (1971) stated,

> Psychotherapy takes place in the overlap of two areas of playing, that of the patient and that of the therapist. Psychotherapy has to do with two people playing together. The corollary of this is that where playing is not possible then the work done by the therapist is directed towards bringing the patient from a state of not being able to play into a state of being able to play.

References

Bion, W. R. (1967) *Second Thoughts*, Heinemann, London.
Casement, P. (1985) *On Learning from the Patient*, Routledge Mental Health Series, London.
Gerhardt, S. (2004) *Why Love Matters*, Routledge, London.
Winnicott, D. W. (1971) *Playing and Reality*, Penguin Books, London.
Winnicott, D. W. (1986) *Home Is Where We Start from*, Penguin Books, London.

Chapter 2

Fantasy and lies

The job of psychotherapy sometimes feels a bit like detective work. As psychotherapists we gather 'clues' about what our clients might be struggling with in the here-and-now from what they present to us in sessions. We try to make sense of this information in the context of what we know about their developmental and family history, as well as their social and cultural experiences. Over a number of sessions we acknowledge fragments of 'evidence' that might not make very much sense to us, or to our client, in isolation. We hold these fragments in mind, rather like metaphorical jigsaw pieces, until we are able to co-create a clearer picture about what might be going on for the young person. But unlike traditional detective work, I would caution that psychotherapy is not a search for empirical truth. Sometimes our clients' narrative is more fantasy than reality – and that's ok. Whatever and however a child or young person communicates with us, they are still sharing something about their external and/or internal world. I am using the term reality rather than truth, and fantasy rather than lie with deliberate intention. As a psychotherapist I am not an arbiter of the truth, in the sense that I neither need nor want to know the accuracy of a young person's narrative. Whatever they present is real for them, even if it is a complete fantasy. My aim in working with children and young people is to help them to unravel the many and varied realities they bring to therapy. These can include lived experiences, as well as conscious and unconscious fears and fantasies, or unconscious *phantasies* as Melanie Klein (1955) called them, which are quite distinct from lies. I think that fantasies can function in a similar way to dreams in that they allow unconscious latent desires and anxieties to become manifest in a more tangible form. Similarly, play, art and creative activities may be used by children and young people to express themselves in a way that words sometimes fail to do. These are more palpable vehicles for carrying unconscious fantasies into the realm of conscious awareness and they are valuable forms of communication. Most adults realise the value of play and art forms as vehicles of expression and exploration. I think that this awareness can be used as a basis for thinking about so-called lies. For example, it would be extremely unlikely, even in the non-therapeutic world, for a young person recounting their dream to be branded a liar or for a child's painting to be labelled a lie. Just as the dream or drawing symbolises and communicates something about the internal world, the young person's spoken fantasy also contains a form or fragment of reality that originates in real, rather than imagined, experience. If we think about fantasies in the same way as we think about other forms of unconscious communication it seems just as ludicrous, I hope, to dismiss them as lies. As with the distinction between content and process, I am interested in how the narrative feels, the emotion it evokes, the way it is told and understood, rather than whether it did or did not happen exactly as it is being told. I then explore with a young person the sense I make, or not, of what they present and see where that takes us. If I were to dismiss their account as a lie, that would be the end of it: game over.

Sometimes a child or adolescent is referred to therapy specifically because someone has deemed him or her to be a liar. They may have been accused, by a parent, carer or professional, of 'making it up' or 'attention-seeking' and the therapist is assigned the wholly inappropriate task of getting them to stop. My baseline is that children and young people need us to listen to what they say, be the content of their narrative reality or fantasy, and that there are usually fragments of one in the other. Psychotherapy is not about 'fixing' the lying client. Instead it is about exploring the meaning of the young person's discourse and helping them to make sense of it. When an adult dismisses a young person's words as lies, they dismiss the young person too and forego an opportunity to communicate with them, both in the here-and-now and in the future. The young person learns that the adult is not interested in what they have to say and so they stop talking to them.

Kelsey

I once had a referral from a social worker who claimed that the adolescent he was supporting merited a diagnosis of pseudologia fantasica. This is an unusual 'diagnosis', first suggested in the medical world around the turn of the twentieth century, to describe patients who told obvious and extreme lies that were perceived by the patients themselves as reality. Although pseudologia fantasica is not recognized as a diagnosable disorder in the Diagnostic Statistical Manual for Mental Disorders, it has warranted discussion in relation to other disorders such as fabricated or induced illness and personality disorders. The key characteristics that had piqued the social worker's attention were that the adolescent – pseudologue – presented endless stories – fantasies – that were detailed and creative but, he declared, totally made up. What also concerned him was that the young person did not appear to have any conscious motive, and at times appeared to be delusional in that she believed her own lies. I was intrigued.

I immediately warmed to thirteen-year-old Kelsey. She was quirky, smart, engaging and engageable. In session one, I invited her to tell me something about herself so I could begin to get to know her. She said she was living with a foster family because her mother was dead and her father was in prison because he had killed her baby sister. She recounted in detail the night of the murder. Kelsey told me she was hiding in a wardrobe in her baby sister's bedroom. Her father was in a rage because he'd had a bad day at work and baby Kenzie would not stop crying. He picked her up and screamed at her to be quiet which only made her cry louder. Kelsey described herself peeking through a crack in the wardrobe door, holding her breath so that her father would not notice she was there and turn his rage towards her. She said she watched silently and terrified as he shook baby Kenzie and hit her repeatedly until she fell quiet and lifeless. Kelsey described seeing blood all over her sister's clothes and dripping from the cot she lay in. She told me that she watched as police officers attended and took her father away, then the ambulance came and took Kenzie, and finally the social worker arrived and took Kelsey. As with most new referrals for looked after children, I had received a preliminary report that provided details of Kelsey's family background and reasons for her being in care. It contained nothing about a sister, a murder or a dead mother. I listened to Kelsey's account and commented that it sounded like a terrifying experience. She agreed that it was, and that she knew she had to remain hidden and quiet to save her own life. She told me that she felt guilty for not protecting her baby sister and I wondered aloud what she could have done. She said she could have stabbed her father with a knife. I worked with Kelsey for a year and she spoke about her sister frequently. She made paintings of the baby's headstone and sang the songs that she said were sung at her funeral. Taken at face value, Kelsey's narrative was a sophisticated and somewhat disturbing lie. However, her fantasy was also a powerful communication about her experience of family life, her sense of murderousness towards a rageful father, of maternal loss and loneliness in a family unable to take care of her as a baby and young infant. I listened, and I commented on the feelings.

After some months I began to share with Kelsey that I was having difficulty making sense of the things she told me about her family. I wondered aloud if maybe things didn't make much sense to her either. One day she came to therapy in an agitated state and said she had something 'really big' to tell me. She said that she didn't have a sister; Kenzie had not been killed because she had never been born! I repeated back that Kelsey had been thinking all this time about the sister who had not been born and how lonely she had felt without an alive baby sibling. I think that Kenzie also represented baby Kelsey – it was interesting that the name she chose sounded so similar to her own. I commented that she seemed to have been thinking about her violent father who she perceived as capable of murder and the mother who she felt was unable to protect her from him. This freed Kelsey up to talk about her experience of domestic violence and neglect, the real experiences that had been tangled up in the fantasy narrative. Had I responded differently, let Kelsey know that I didn't believe her, or opted for a tentative diagnostic label, I would have denied her the opportunity to reflect on her feelings and make sense of her experiences.

Harvey

Like Kelsey, Harvey's narrative was both enduring and fantastical. He was referred to me for psychotherapy aged nine following concerns about his behaviour at school in the context of possible safeguarding issues. Harvey came to the attention of the behaviour management team following a number of playground scuffles, having previously remained under their radar. At this point, that is, once he had the attention of people in authority and the opportunity to be listened to, Harvey disclosed that his mother was in hospital with a terrible disease that caused her to lapse in and out of consciousness. Harvey was upset because his father was 'mean' and would not allow him to visit his mother and he really missed her. A meeting between home and school easily disproved Harvey's version of events and confirmed that his mother was home and physically well. However, his mother did acknowledge to the school's family liaison officer (FLO) that there was some 'tension' in the family and she also admitted that she had felt depressed since the birth of her second child, Harvey's little sister, Harriet. Harvey's mother consented to the suggestion of a referral for a psychological intervention for Harvey and also agreed to speak to her doctor to request mental health support for herself. I received a telephone referral from the FLO and met with her for a consultation to think about Harvey. I agreed to work with him in school because this seemed the best option logistically. My main point of contact remained the FLO rather than Harvey's parents, neither of whom I met.

When I first encountered Harvey I was struck by how small he was for a Year 5 child. He seemed both physically underweight and emotionally vulnerable, and I perceived him as a 'little boy'. I told Harvey that I had been asked to meet with him because his teachers thought he had been acting differently to usual and that they had become concerned about him. He told me he had been in trouble for fighting and that he had 'kicked Ashley's head in'. I said that sounded like he might be feeling angry and he nodded and said that he was. I wondered if he had any thoughts about where his anger might be coming from and he said,

From my dad; my dad makes me angry because he won't let me see my mum.

I responded to the communication about how Harvey was feeling,

You're feeling angry with your dad...

rather than the story around it. Harvey told me that his mum had been sick for a long time and that she was 'terminal' which made him really sad. I agreed that when someone close to us is sick it is very ordinary to feel sad. I wanted not only to acknowledge and validate his feelings but also to unpick them, so I added that we might feel sad both for the person who is sick and also for ourselves. Harvey picked up on this and said he was sad for himself because his mother had not been able to make him nice dinners since she had been sick like she used to before, and now he has to get his own, or eat what his dad made which was mostly cold beans on toast. I repeated back to Harvey that things felt different at home now to how they used to be before. I also remembered aloud that he had mentioned his mum had been sick for a long time and I wondered when he had first noticed this. He said it was when he came to school, and when his sister was born. I acknowledged out load that there was a lot going on around that time; Harvey started school, his baby sister was born and his mum got sick. I said it must have felt as if everything was changing. Harvey he said 'it sucked' and he stuck his thumb in his mouth, both as if to unconsciously illustrate sucking as well as in an attempt to self-soothe. He told me that he only went to the hospital once and that all the nurses were really nice. He remembered a male nurse in particular who let Harvey choose a sweet from a jar on the nurse's station but his sister wasn't allowed to have one because she was, 'just a baby who had just been born'. I wondered aloud how old Harvey was then, maybe about five, and he nodded.

I had a sense that Harvey's change in behaviour as he entered school Year 5 symbolised something of the changes he experienced when he was five years old. It was a fact that Harvey's mother went to hospital, not because she was sick, but to give birth to his sister, and that this significant event coincided with another: his starting school. It seemed to me that Harvey was re-experiencing his earlier experiences of maternal separation so powerfully that it felt to him as if they were happening in the here-and-now. The birth of a sibling can create a trauma for the child who, until such time, has been the sole occupant of his mother's preoccupation. Hospitals can be confusing places for children to contemplate. They may have heard about sick people going there, sometimes to get better but at other times to die or disappear for good. Often, well-meaning families prohibit children from visiting their inpatient relatives, as Harvey's father did, and so hospitals come to represent frightening places that keep them from their loved ones. For children, the fantasy they create in their minds is often much more terrifying than the reality, if only it had been explained. When Harvey was five his mother was taken to hospital where she remained for five days, coinciding with his first week of primary school. Thought about in context, Harvey's claim that his mother was suffering from a terminal illness illustrates his unbearable fear that their separation would be forever. My knowledge of the school curriculum provided further context that helped me to make sense of Harvey's fantasy. Year 5 involves much discussion about the impending move to secondary school. Children go on transition day visits and some of them sit tests to help select which secondary school they will attend. I think that all this talk about starting a new school had triggered something for Harvey about the experience of starting his new primary school and how distressing that time had been for him. Harvey's internal world seemed to have become a confusing tangle of illness, babies, separation and loss. His assertion that his mother had contracted 'a terrible disease' seemed symbolic of his internal reality. My hypothesis was that the 'terrible disease' denoted pregnancy and birth. Not surprisingly, Harvey had experienced feelings of rejection as his mother's attention shifted from him to her new baby. His mother had also reported feeling depressed, post-natally and still, three years later. For Harvey, it must have felt as if she was 'in and out of consciousness'.

Psychoanalytic theory suggests that, at some level, even very young children associate pregnancy and birth with the 'primal scene' – that is the occasion on which they first become aware of their parents' sexual intercourse – and that this is often experienced as aggressive and frightening (Freud, 1918). Harvey depicted his father as 'mean', while mother reported 'tension' in the marital relationship. Had Harvey reconciled this parental 'tension' with the sexual act that produced the baby? Perhaps. Furthermore, Harvey's assertion that his father was 'mean' was illustrated by the embargo on visits to see mother in hospital. In other words, his meanness was exemplified by his standing in the way of the relationship between mother and son in order to keep his wife to himself. According to Freudian theory, this all occurred at a crucial age for Harvey, during the Oedipal stage of development. His lived experience coincides with the arousal of an unconscious desire for the mother and a wish to exclude the father, who is perceived as excluding *him* from the parental relationship. From an Oedipal perspective, Harvey's father was vilified – he was described as 'mean' – but because Harvey could not fight his father, his anger was displaced and he 'kicked Ashley's head in'. The Oedipal stage of development is also when children's awareness of sexual difference is heightened, which can bring about both speculation and fear. I had no direct knowledge of how Harvey responded to his new baby sibling, a girl without a penis, but I am certain he would have wondered about the differences between them. I am aware that many people struggle with Freudian theory, dismissing it as fantastical and with an overemphasis on infantile sexuality. For me, the complete works of Freud provided the keystone of my learning about psychodynamic psychotherapy and they continue to influence my thinking and for-mulations two decades on. Freud's theories certainly helped inform my hypotheses in relation to Harvey's 'fantasies'. It was possible, over time, for Harvey to work through his overwhelming feelings of love, hate and rejection in therapy. His emotional responses were undoubtedly real. The fantasy narrative he presented was simply a way to make those feelings manifest, and a vehicle to carry them into conscious awareness so that they could be listened to, thought about and made sense of.

Sexual abuse

In my clinical experience, what has been dismissed as a lie usually contains fragments of reality. In many cases, these realities relate to current or historical abuse. The obvious hypothesis on these occasions is that disbelief is a more comfortable position than the intolerable re-ality and unbearable-ness of child abuse. In deciding that a young per-son's allegation of abuse is a lie, the network around them can avoid thinking about it further because they have made up their mind that it did not happen. This is a classic illustration of denial as a form of ego defence: denying the abuse, and therefore not thinking about it. It is also a way to avoid becoming enmeshed in it. Working with sexu-ally abused young people can sometimes feel risky and it always feels messy. The messy narrative gets told in a messy way, either verbally or non-verbally, and we are often left with a physical mess in the room and a psychological mess in our minds. Children and young people who have been sexually abused have messy internal worlds. They can-not comprehend their reality any more than we can and so sometimes they create a fantasy, either as a means of escape, or in an effort to make sense of their experiences. These fantasies deserve to be listened to so that the young people have a little less mess to carry around.

Online fantasy

Many of the children and young people I meet in therapy have grown up in homes where boundaries are, at best, permeable. Many have witnessed aggression and violence, directly or indirectly, and many have experienced trauma, neglect and abuse. Without bound-aries to protect them and to separate their self from others, these children feel unsafe, unheld and uncared for. Not surprisingly, re-search suggests that they are twice as likely as those who have not experienced adverse childhood experiences to develop a formal mental illness. A lack of boundaries in the external world can result in a merging of the boundary between reality and fantasy. As a means of escape, many children and young people retreat into a fantasy world provided by console games. In doing so, they form identifications with online fantasy characters who are fighters, killers and abusers. Such identifications form a defence against their own vulnerabilities and their own experiences of being attacked or abused. For some children, the violent fantasy worlds they withdraw to online mirror their external lives so that fantasy and reality become tangled up. What they play and act out feels real, and what they experience in the real world feels no different. Such games remain popular with pre-adolescent and adolescent boys who,

...crave raw, loud and angry...because they need it to be strong enough to match and master their [own] anxiety and anger.

(Jones, 2002)

Many of the boys and young men whom I meet in therapy lack a good enough male role model, either because of a real absence of a father or because their father figures are inconsistent or abusive. Once again, the online fantasy world provides an opportunity to fill the gap in the process of identity formation. Boys who have grown up without a good enough father figure, become enmeshed with on-screen characters who present an exaggerated version of themselves (Taransaud, 2011).

Paige

Eleven-year-old Paige insisted she was a mermaid. She told me that the reason I couldn't see her mermaid tail was because it only grew when she got wet below the waist. She said that the rest of the time she could pretend she was normal and go around on legs looking like everyone else. Paige had complex learning difficulties and global developmental delay. It was hypothesised that her difficulties were a result of trauma and severe neglect, both pre-natal and post-birth. Paige was a looked after child in specialist therapeutic foster care who had been emotionally, physically and sexually abused by her mother. Maternal sexual abuse remains the ultimate unthinkable act. Paige could not think about it either and so she created the mermaid fantasy as a psychological defence. Much of the abuse occurred when Paige was pre-verbal, meaning that her memories were pre-verbal too. She literally did not have the words to describe her experiences, but that did not mean that she had no memories of them, even though the memories were mostly at an unconscious or preconscious level and also, I think, contained within her body. Paige's mermaid fantasy delivered a sophisticated communication that, once listened to, enabled her to make some sense of herself.

One social care report stated that, as an infant, Paige had been regularly left in saturated nappies for days and that on one unannounced visit from social care her cot was discovered covered in faeces. This meant that she had spent the majority of her infancy 'wet below the waist'. As an eleven-year-old, Paige displayed poor hygiene and struggled to manage menstruation, which served to replicate her early experience. I suspected that reinventing herself as a mermaid was a way of defending herself against this disgusting reality. I told Paige, honestly, that I did not know much about mermaids but that I was interested to learn. She responded with a huge grin and said that everyone else told her that mermaids were not real and that she was just being silly to think that they were. She said that *no-one* had *ever* wanted to talk to her about mermaids before! I said, honestly, that I did not think she was silly and that I really wanted to hear what she had to say. Paige was excited and asked what I wanted to know. I suggested that we start at the beginning and that I was wondering if mermaids were born as mermaids or whether ordinary people grow into mermaids later. Paige said that she was a mermaid because her mother gave her crushed pearls and seawater when she was a baby. I believe that this fantasy contained fragments of Paige's lived experience. The social care report stated that her mother abused substances during her pregnancy and in the years following Paige's birth. My hypothesis was that Paige had made a symbolic association between the cocaine and alcohol she was known to have ingested in utero and the magical mermaid potion of 'crushed pearls and seawater' that she found more palatable. I acknowledged her belief that her mother had made her the way that she was from what she had given her to eat. There appeared to be some truth in the fantasy.

Although I really did not know much about mermaids, what I did know was that they had ambiguous genitalia. I asked Paige about this in developmentally appropriate language,

How do you know if mermaids are boys or girls?

She told me it was obvious,

Mermaids are girls because they are *maids*.

She added that,

Boy mermaids are called mer*boys*.

I said I had never heard of a merboy before but that the word made sense. Paige said that she hadn't heard of them either until she said it! She was evidently confused about boys and girls and about the differences between them. How could she be anything *but* confused about gender and sex? All that she could know for sure was that her own female body had brought a lifetime of suffering: sexual abuse, maternal-neglect and self-neglect. No wonder she wanted to deny the very existence of it by choosing to ignore the reality of her developing body and replacing it with a fishy appendage in lieu of female genitalia. I think that the mermaid's tail communicated something else about Paige's reality: a disbelief in her capacity to stand on her own two feet. Thought about in the context of her developmental history, Paige's identification as a mermaid symbolised her incomprehensible sense of self as she waivered on the threshold of adolescence. For her, the fantasy was real because it contained fragments of memory and relics of lived experience. The pretence for her was that she was 'normal and could go around looking like everyone else'.

Maurice

Maurice was a twelve-year-old boy who had reportedly suffered familial sexual abuse as an infant. He and his young, single mother shared a home with his maternal aunt and her two children, a son and a daughter. The details were sketchy, but it was believed that Maurice's male cousin had forced Maurice to perform masturbation when he was about four, and his cousin was around twelve. The adolescent's mother, Maurice's aunt, dismissed her nephew's disclosure outright and deemed Maurice to be a liar. His own mother had difficulty contemplating the 'unthinkable' and struggled to comfort her son. Relationships within the family home became strained until eventually Maurice was sent to live with his maternal grandmother who took on the role of legal guardian when he was aged seven.

Maurice was referred to me for a therapeutic assessment not long after the transition to secondary school. Teachers observed that he was subdued in the classroom, while in the playground he would often get into fights and was observed to be manipulative. I met Maurice for an initial assessment with his grandmother who warned me that,

> While he might have the face of an angel, he lies like the devil.

I heard that Maurice was struggling at school, both academically and socially, and that his grandmother didn't know what to do with him. I thought he deserved to be listened to. Maurice turned up to therapy each week under his own steam, as it was a short walk from where he went to school. He didn't say much but invited me to play board games. He selected games of luck rather than skill and the sessions didn't feel particularly playful; in fact they felt like a bit of a drudge. Maurice and I had been meeting for about a month when his grandmother got in touch to tell me about a screwed up piece of paper she had found in Maurice's bedroom. On it was a drawing of one boy, labelled Maurice, performing oral sex on another boy, labelled Anton. Grandmother identified Anton as a neighbour and a 'good boy' who was a similar age to Maurice. She told me that she was absolutely certain nothing 'untoward' had happened between them and that she was informing me about the note so that I could 'address the lying'. One of the things that struck me was that his grandmother appeared either unwilling or unable to talk with Maurice about her discovery. Grandmother's belief in the 'good' boy set up an effective split between bad/abuse and good/non-abuse. She also appeared reluctant to *think*, instead opting to get rid of her thoughts by giving them to me to deal with. This is not uncommon in families where there has been an experience of child sexual abuse, which is perhaps the epitome of unthinkable. But by splitting it off, the young person becomes split-off and unthinkable-about too. He or she becomes the child who is forced out of home, excluded from school and/or branded a liar. I had to bear in mind all of the possible realities and bear witness to whatever was given to me to think about.

I reflected on this new information in the context of Maurice's unresolved (alleged) childhood abuse and wondered if and how the two could be related. I was mindful that history might be repeating itself in terms of a sexually abusive experience, but in the very least, I could be certain that Maurice was re-experiencing disbelief from the maternal figure responsible for looking after him. I was also conscious of the fact that Maurice and Anton were both aged twelve, the age of Maurice's cousin when the alleged incident took place. It was vital for me to provide Maurice with a space to think, alongside someone who was prepared to think with him.

The next time we met, Maurice demonstrated his availability for symbolic thinking quite beautifully using the sand tray. The sand was damp and had formed lumps that Maurice crumbled between his fingers to get rid of. He offered me a plastic rake so that I could join him in the sand without get my hands dirty. I commented that he seemed to want my help in raking things up and also that he had a desire to protect me and keep me clean. I held the rake in my right hand and slowly moved the lumpy sand around in the tray. With my left hand I sprinkled the soft grains, illustrating that I didn't mind getting my hands in the sand with my client. In his own time and without any prompting from me, Maurice told me that he had been 'forced to do something'. I said that it sounded difficult for him to talk about, and that from his facial expression perhaps it was something he found disgusting. Maurice nodded. In lieu of naming the sex act he gagged and told me it had made him feel sick. He said he wanted it to stay a secret because thinking about it made him want to puke. I reminded Maurice that I would listen to anything he wanted to say here, even the disgusting stuff, and that while it would remain a private space, sometimes secrets needed to be shared in order to keep young people safe. Maurice told me that he had been thinking about something that happened to him a long time ago, that he had told his family about but they hadn't believed him, and that he had not talked about it with anyone since. I believe that Maurice's difficulty in naming his experience was mirrored in his family, which felt 'gagged' and unable to acknowledge something as sickening as childhood sexual abuse. Maintaining my position *alongside* rather than being *drawn in* was not easy, but it afforded me the emotional distance and perspective that Maurice needed me to provide in order for him to feel contained and attended to. Alice Miller (1998) suggests that a therapist should,

> ...devote his full attention as a spectator to the drama, without jumping onto the stage and joining in the act.

I told Maurice that it was not my role to investigate the facts, but that perhaps I could help him to process his thoughts and feelings about what had happened, so that it didn't feel so hard and dis-gusting in his head. He seemed relieved and continued to talk. He told me he had pushed it to the side of his head 'where the bad stuff is' so that he could focus on the 'good stuff'. Maurice did not elaborate, but as he talked he continued to shift the sand between his fingers. After a while I noticed that one half of the sand tray contained finely sifted sand while the 'hard bits' or symbolic 'bad stuff' had been separated to the other side. When I commented on this, Maurice said that was exactly what it was like inside his head. His sand play provided a concrete illustration of his attempt to split off the trauma as well as, perhaps, his family's attempt to deny it by pushing it aside. Because I had been able to think with Maurice, rather than question his motives, and because I had demonstrated my availability to listen to him, rather than deny his reality, he had been able to communicate his feelings more coherently. I think that what I witnessed was what Winnicott (1967) described as the,

> ...space between inner world and outer reality [which] creates the possibility for playing and for the filling of the space with symbols.

In contrast, Maurice's family remained fixed in their belief that he was a liar. I attempted to encourage his grandmother to think with and about Maurice and to encourage him to talk to her. Instead she questioned him and interpreted his confusion as lies and confirma-tion that he could not be trusted. Clinical research with children who have experienced trauma or abuse suggests that doubt and confusion is evidence of attempts to recall a true memory rather than of inventing a lie (Mordock, 2001). I suggested to Maurice's grandmother that he was trying to make sense of his experiences and that his graphic representation of oral sex with a peer was likely to contain (at least) fragments of reality. I commented on the timing of the drawings; Maurice and Anton were both aged twelve, the same age as Maurice's cousin at the time of the alleged inci-dent. His grandmother dismissed this as coincidence. I continued to work with Maurice for a year, exploring his ordinary adolescent sexual development in the context of memories of sexually abusive experiences. This was mostly at a symbolic level through sand play and drawings, which I witnessed and was curious about.

Many children and young people have been accused of telling lies. What I have discovered in listening to them is that they are often confused, frightened and traumatised. Psychoanalytic theory can help us to reflect upon so-called lies and reframe them as fantasies, which are simply vehicles of symbolic communication. Children's fantasies are always autobiographical. They contain disguised and fragmented aspects of internal and external realities that are too overwhelming in their original form. It is our role, as adults, to listen with a sensitive and open mind, rather than react in a punitive or disbelieving way. I think this is true whomever a child confides in, be it parent/carer, therapist or other professional. It is a valuable experience to be thought *about* and thought *with*, an experience, which, of course, is fundamental to therapy. However, I believe that any adult can enhance communication with a child or young person by taking on board some of what psychodynamic thinking has taught us. And the most fundamental thing is to *listen* and to avoid the temptation to dismiss a young person's discourse as a lie.

References

Diagnostic and Statistical Manual of Mental Disorders (DSM-V) (2013) American Psychiatric Association.

Freud, S. (1918) *The Standard Edition of the Complete Psychological Works of Sigmund Freud, Volume XVII* (1917–1919): An Infantile Neurosis and Other Works, pp. 1–124, Vintage Publishing, London.

Jones, G. (2002) *Killing Monsters: Why Children Need Fantasy, Super-Heroes and Make-Believe Violence*, Basic Books, New York.

Klein, M. (1955) 'The psycho-analytic play technique: Its history and significance', In Klein, M. Heimann, P., and Money-Kyrle, R. E. (eds.), *New Directions in Psycho-Analysis*, Tavistock Publications, London.

Miller, A. (1998) 'Two psychoanalytic approaches' (p. 16). In *Thou Shalt Not Be Aware*, Pluto Press, London.

Mordock, J. B. (2001) 'Interviewing abused and traumatized children', *Clinical Child Psychology and Psychiatry* 6 (2), 271–291, Sage, London.

Taransaud, D. (2011) *You Think I'm Evil*, Worth Publishing, London.

Winnicott, D. (1967) 'Mirror-role of mother and family in child development', In *Playing and Reality*, Winnicott, D. (1971), Penguin, London.

Chapter 3

Labelling children and young people

The proclivity for labelling children and young people continues to flourish, as does the debate about whether or not this is helpful. For me the question is less about *how* helpful it is to label, and more about *whom* the label serves to help. I also think that the issue of labelling is related to judgement. Like all language, these terms are subjective. Within the medical, educational and, to a lesser extent, therapeutic arenas, labelling seems to be a widely accepted outcome of assessment and diagnosis. It is something that professionals do to non-professionals. Labelling has therefore been perceived, on the whole, as a 'good thing'. Judgement, on the other hand, can be done by anyone, to anyone and has largely been perceived as a 'bad thing'. Most children are taught, from a very young age, that it is wrong to judge others. They are also taught that they must be wary of strangers, choose friends who are 'appropriate' and later on make similar choices regarding romantic, sexual and life partners and perhaps even counsellors or therapists. How can children and young people make discerning choices about the people they encounter without judging them? I think the simple answer is they cannot. To tell a child or young person not to judge other people is to tell them to ignore human instinct and intuition that has evolved over millennia. If we relate to others indiscriminately, without judgement, we would not survive for very long. This ill-informed advice is doled out beyond the sphere of parenting. From what I hear anecdotally, the edict of many counsellor trainings appears to be something along the lines of 'thou shalt not judge'. I think it is ludicrous to demand that trainees deny their instincts in order to take up, in my opinion, a wholly inappropriate, non-judgemental position. Of course counsellors and therapists judge, even those who profess that they do not. We judge our peers, supervisors and trainers – how else can we decide who is best placed to teach us? We judge what we read, what we hear and what we see – how else can we learn from our experiences? And yes, we judge our clients – how else can we contemplate their needs? We might call it 'therapeutic assessment' but judgement by another name is still judgement. Judgement is a theme that rears its head a lot in my therapeutic practice. Parents and carers feel judged on their capacity as parents, on the choices they make about work/life balance and on their social status. Children sense they are being judged on their popularity among their peers, on their appearance, on the stuff that they have or do not have. And adolescents think they are being judged on... well on *absolutely everything by absolutely everyone*. Adolescents often tell me they feel 'paranoid' and what they mean by that is that they feel as if people are looking at them and judging them. I don't tell them they are over-reacting. I don't tell them they are wrong. I don't refer them to a psychiatrist for assessment and diagnostic labelling because the truth is, they *are* being looked at and they *are* being judged. Judging is part of the human condition and, because I'm human too, it's also part of therapy. For me, clinical judgement is an important therapeutic responsibility. I remain carefully attuned to a depressed mother so that I can make a judgement about her capacity to care for her children. To be non-judgemental would mean disregarding what I witness and ignoring my felt sense of what is going on for the family. This would be both unethical and immoral. I have an obligation to safeguard the children and young people I work with and sometimes that involves making a judgement about their family environment. When the mother accuses me of judging her, I can say honestly that I have been wondering if she can be a good enough mother at a time when her own struggles are so overwhelming. She might still feel judged, she has probably been judging (and berating) herself too, but she also feels noticed and cared about. Much of my work with adolescents includes making a judgement about risk. Young people tell me about their consumption of drugs and alcohol, about underage or promiscuous sex, and about self-injury. I don't judge their choices, but I do make judgements about their capacity to keep themselves safe and I share these with the young people in sessions. If I didn't, how would they know that I had noticed what they had shared with me and how would they know that I cared? I am sometimes asked to share my clinical judgements in meetings and court reports where decisions are made about children's welfare. I share my judgements honestly and always with the families involved before anyone else. Do these families feel judged? Of course they do, but I assure them that my role is to help to make sense of their situation and communicate their needs so that they are able to access the support they deserve.

Every therapeutic encounter invites multiple hypotheses about a client's state of mind, as well as their wishes, feelings, experiences and needs. Therapists are trained to analyse the client's narrative, conscious and unconscious, said and unsaid, and what is analysis if not a type of judgement? I think that to be judged is to be noticed and that is what I hope to convey to the children, young people and families I work with. When someone tells me that they feel judged, either by their peers, parents, me or the world at large, I do not try to cajole them our of it or fool them into believing that I am non-judgemental. Instead I share my judgements honestly and transparently. I want them to know that I judge them because I have noticed them and had a feeling response to them.

The way that labelling has been differentiated from judgement sets up a number of good/bad splits, such as professional/non-professional and acceptable/unacceptable. Splitting is never helpful; it ignores the nuances of reality and stops us from thinking. To take the case in point, it also serves to maintain a hierarchy – an 'us and them' – and this amplifies the power imbalance between 'knowing' therapist and 'unknowing' client which is not helpful either. I think it is beneficial to unpick and reframe the way labelling is used in relation to therapeutic work. A diagnostic label can serve as a shortcut to explaining behaviour. If a young person is referred to me with a label of Attention Deficit Hyperactivity Disorder (ADHD), for example, I might *think* I know what to expect. The young person, probably male, is likely to be fidgety, with difficulties affecting their concentration, engagement and/or learning. Adults in their lives might perceive them as rude, angry and aggressive. They are probably underachieving academically and struggling socially. Previous generations, in an era before widespread diagnostic labelling, might have described the young person as 'naughty' or 'unmanageable'. Adults would have been more likely to suggest 'a clip around the ear' or other corporal punishment rather than medication and/or therapy. I have met many young people who match the stereotype of their ADHD label. I have also met those for whom the label acts as a self-fulfilling prophecy,

I've got ADHD so I'll behave like I've got ADHD

which might be conscious or it might not. The ADHD stereotype, like any other, only partially explains the young person's reality and fails to acknowledge the idiosyncrasies of the individual as a whole. I have also met young people with a label of ADHD who have learnt to manage their inattention and channel their hyperactivity in order to achieve. I have met others still who do not match the criteria of the label they have been given in any way at all.

Felix

I had a referral from a professional woman, Vonny, who was struggling to manage her son's behaviour. I met with her to think through her experience of mothering. Vonny told me she had wanted to be a mother for her entire adult life. She had suffered a number of miscarriages in her mid and late thirties in the context of a long-term heterosexual relationship. When the relationship ended, not long after Vonny's fortieth birthday, she thought she would have to relinquish the hope of ever becoming a mother. This was something Vonny found too heart breaking to contemplate and she took the decision to conceive via a surrogate. Vonny gave birth to Felix when she was forty-five and was raising him as a working lone-parent. When I wondered about Vonny's own experience of being mothered, she described her childhood not only as 'fairly traditional' but also as 'less than ideal'. She told me that her father went out to work, while her mother stayed at home to look after her and her younger brother. She recalled a 'shouty dad' and a 'placid mum' with little affection shown either within the martial relationship or between parents and children. As Vonny was talking about her desire to be a mother, I was struck by the love and yearning she had seemed to carry for her yet-to-be-born child. For her 'entire adult life' she had created a fantasy of herself as a mother and of the child or children she would co-create within a happy, stable relationship. It was also evident that, in her fantasy, her constructed family would be very different to the one she had grown up in and that her own child would receive an abundance of love. When we began to talk about the present, and about Vonny's concerns for Felix, something shifted. She bristled slightly and said she thought he probably had ADHD. She wanted to know if I could offer him anger management and suggest some behavioural techniques to settle him down. I asked Vonny to give me an idea about what Felix was like. She said he was never still, always racing around the place and climbing the walls. She said he would not sleep, was always hungry and always on the go. She admitted that any efforts on her part to curtail him were met with opposition and defiance. Vonny admitted she was at her wit's end and didn't know what to do.

I should point out at this stage, now that you have an image of Felix, that he had recently turned three when this conversation took place. I had a strong sense that Vonny felt disappointed; in herself as a mother or in Felix her son I was not quite sure. What seemed painfully evident though was that Vonny's reality had not matched up to her long-held fantasy of motherhood. I suggested it might be helpful for us to meet again and for her to bring Felix along too so that we could think about him together some more. Vonny agreed and a week later she brought Felix to meet me. Felix was a delight! He curiously poked his nose and his fingers into my cupboards and drawers, pulled books from shelves and toys from boxes. I commented on how keen he seemed to explore, while also modelling containment with phrases such as,

> There are things in this room that are private and I'd like you not to touch them.

I guided him away from what I'd rather he not touch, and towards the things he might enjoy instead,

> Why don't we see what's inside this toy box...?

Felix chatted away, sometimes to himself, sometimes narrating his play but also asking endless questions of me. He responded in an age-appropriate way, by pushing the boundaries but also staying within them once he realised they was firm. We spent the entire session like this, with Vonny witnessing me, observing, responding to and joining in with Felix. Towards the end of the session I turned my attention back to Vonny and commended her on her bright and inquisitive little boy. She expressed her relief that there was nothing 'wrong' with her son and admitted her anxieties about not being a good mum. Felix didn't need a label. He needed his mother to be acknowledged and offered containment so that she could acknowledge and contain her little boy. It is difficult to feel as if you are a good enough mother, if you have had little experience of being mothered yourself.

Why label?

Young people with labels are sometimes stereotypical and sometimes self-fulfilling. Some buck the trend while others leave me feeling perplexed as to why the label was ever assigned to them in the first place. My confusion often mirrors confusion elsewhere, in the system or parent, as was the case with Vonny and Felix. The good thing about the diagnostic criteria for Autistic Spectrum Condition (ASC), compared with some other labels, is that it recognises the condition as a spectrum. I would argue that the whole gamut of ordinary and disordered behaviour lies somewhere along a continuum. Children and young people oscillate up and down various spectrums depending on their age and developmental capacity, context and mood. As do all of us. On any given day any one of them could be labelled with some disorder or other but it does not mean that they *should* be or that it would be helpful. Labels are usually assigned from unfamiliar professionals based on a snapshot of observed behaviour. What that means is that on that particular day the young person met that particular set of criteria. On a different day in a different mood and context, even with a different professional, they might, and probably would, behave and be labelled differently. So with so many ifs, buts and maybes, what is the point in labelling? For many, a label is a ticket that allows access to treatment and support from health, therapeutic or specialist education provisions. There is little wonder then that they are prized (and in some cases 'priced') so dearly.

A more controversial aspect of labelling is that it can be seen as a way to let people off the hook. If a child is labelled with ADHD they are not naughty or unmanageable, or a consequence of an uncontaining environment; they are *disordered*. If a young person has a label of ASC they are not rude and antisocial; they have a *condition*. If they have a label of Oppositional Defiance Disorder (ODD) they are not the stubborn and wilful product of indulgent parenting; they cannot help it. A label deems both parent and child blameless. I have met countless families that have struggled for years finally making improvements after their child has been labelled. But it is not the label that makes the difference. It is access to the right type of support, based on an understanding of the child or young person's needs. The label might provide the shortcut, the headline about their behaviour or the entry ticket into services, but listening to the young person and thinking about them holistically is what really makes the difference.

Child and adolescent mental health professionals, including psychologists, counsellors and psychotherapists, receive a huge number of referrals of violent and aggressive boys (in particular) who are unable to concentrate, are failing academically and have no impulse control. In many cases, the boys have been unofficially labelled ADHD. Another bunch of young people, again usually boys, are described as lacking in empathy, obsessional, hypervigilant and overly sensitive. They are frequently thought of as 'on the spectrum'. Often, a mental health diagnosis is sought by the referrer in order to explain the child or young person's behaviour and, in many cases they are also seeking a drug to control it. I recognise and support thoughtful, accurate diagnosis and treatment, but to label someone without sufficient thought, care and understanding is tantamount to imposing a hypothetical version of reality onto an already confused young person. In my opinion, any mental health assessment is incomplete if we ignore the family and environmental experiences. To do so might result in a neat diagnosis, but it is also likely to leave the child exposed to further risk and potentially irreversible damage.

Bembé

Bembé was a nine-year-old Afro-Caribbean boy who was referred to me for a psychotherapy assessment by his social worker who stated that,

> he meets every single one of the criteria for ADHD.

The referral letter highlighted Bembé's hyperactivity and inattention. It described him as a bully who manipulated and terrorised his peers. It said he used inappropriate sexualised language and behaviour and was verbally and physically aggressive to staff and students alike. At the time of referral, Bembé was on a fixed term exclusion from school for hitting his pregnant primary school teacher with a chair. I met with the social worker and Bembé's mother, Jazz, who appeared to show signs of bruising on her cheek. I was told that Bembé was out of control and needed to be 'tamed'. It sounded to me as if they were describing a wild animal rather than a little boy. On examining the family history, I learnt that Bembé was an unplanned baby, born when Jazz had just turned twenty. His father drank 'to manage his anxiety' and was sometimes 'a bit' aggressive.

Jazz seemed reluctant to elaborate but the social worker told me that Bembé's father was violent throughout the pregnancy and that Jazz gave birth to her first child with a black eye. The family were referred to social services before mother and son were discharged from hospital and had been known to professionals on and off throughout Bembé's life. Jazz told me she had 'made bad choices' regarding men and admitted that each of her partners had been violent and had used drugs or alcohol or both. She had five children under nine, to five different fathers and was in a relationship with Des, the father of her six-month-old baby, at the time we met. When I wondered about her current relationship she told me,

It's ok, you know, normal...

As she trailed off I wondered aloud what she meant by normal; did she mean violent. Jazz said that Des was,

OK really, not as bad as some but admitted that he sometimes knocks me about a bit.

I agreed to meet Bembé for one session to offer my professional opinion as to whether he was likely to meet the criteria for ADHD or whether, as I already suspected, his presentation could be made sense of without labelling.

When I met Bembé I was struck by his size. The image that had been portrayed of him was of a monstrous aggressor yet I perceived him as a small, underweight boy who seemed weak and scrawny, like a little bird that had been pushed from its nest too soon. Bembé seemed interested in the art materials and I invited him to draw a picture so that I could learn a bit about him. He drew a series of stick figures, clumsily in black felt tip pen, under the heading 'family'. His hands were messy and stained with black ink that got rubbed across the page so that it and the family looked grimy and sullied. Bembé told me that his mum was a 'slag' and he drew her pregnant and with a black eye. When I wondered how that had happened, I think I was referring to the pregnancy as well as the beating, he said, 'it was him' and pointed at a looming figure on the page he called Des. Bembé said,

I fucking hate Des and that he wished he would, fuck off and die.

I repeated back that he really fucking hated Des and he looked at me, amazed, and we made a connection. Some professionals do not condone swearing in the presence of nine-year-olds, but I always use their own language to mirror their words and describe their feelings and it seemed important to acknowledge the intensity of the *fucking* hatred. Bembé told me that Des was mean to his mum 'like they all are' and that he had to look after her and make sure she was alright but that he also felt angry with her because it was sort of her own fault that it kept happening. I acknowledged that it seemed as if his mum didn't make safe choices about men and that I could see why that would annoy him and make him feel that he had to take care of her. I wondered how Bembé was able to do that when he was at school all day and he admitted that if he kicked off enough they sent him home. That made a lot of sense of his behaviour. I asked Bembé what he liked to do when he wasn't at school and he told me he played Grand Theft Auto. I wondered aloud what Bembé enjoyed about the game and he said,

> The sex and the killing

the most honest and straightforward answer I think I've ever received to a question like that.

Bembé is illustrative of countless boys (in particular) whose lives are furnished with both real and virtual sex and violence. Their external lives are messy, unsafe and unboundaried and so it is no surprise that their internal worlds are the same and that they present as chaotic, uncontrollable and at risk of exclusion. Children like Bembé,

> ...create havoc at home and school... as if they were spilling out all over the place.
>
> (Jennings, 2011)

I shared my hypothesis with Bembé's social worker and his mother that his presentation seemed to be symbolic of his internalised sense of the world. I said that it seemed to me as if he had swallowed up his experiences and then projected them out quite literally because they didn't make any sense. I likened this to ingesting something poisonous, being unable to digest it and then spewing it out again. They seemed to get it. I also added, just to be clear, that a label of ADHD would be of little benefit and that what Bembé needed instead was to feel safe and contained.

Elijah

As well as an increase in requests for diagnostic labelling, I have also noticed an inclination to label, what I see as, ordinary emotion as something else. I have wondered about the effect of pathologising feelings, medicating and labelling them, rather than acknowledging and feeling them. I have also wondered about the impact for young people of trying to switch off their emotions so that they become robotic and feeling-less – but perhaps more manageable. I received a referral from a local grammar school for seventeen-year-old Elijah. The head of sixth form outlined concerns that the student was depressed and suicidal. I offered him an initial consultation, which he attended alone after school. Elijah was a bright and articulate young man who told me he was confused about the therapy referral but decided to come

To get them off my back.

By 'them' he meant his teachers and parents. I invited Elijah to tell me about what was going on for him. He said he was studying for A' levels and contemplating university options. He had loads of coursework for two of his subjects and mock exams coming up in the other two. He enjoyed school and was hoping to achieve good enough grades to study sport science at a top UK university. Elijah had two part time jobs, as a lifeguard at the local pool and as a sports coach at a summer school. He was clearly a busy young man. I wondered how Elijah managed to juggle all of his commitments and he said he just got on with it and they didn't really feel like commitments because everything he did was through choice. When I wondered if he was struggling with anything, Elijah told me he was struggling with his Universities and Colleges Admissions Service (UCAS) application, particularly with writing his personal statement. We spent most of the session thinking about this – about his strengths, work experience, hobbies and interests. He had got so bogged down in the *doing* that he had been unable to take a step back and observe his many strengths and aptitudes. When I wondered if Elijah had ever done anything to hurt himself, or thought about hurting himself, he looked at me aghast. I told him that his teacher had thought he was depressed and that he might want to die. I wondered aloud where that notion might have come from. I saw the proverbial penny drop as Elijah's facial expression registered the moment. He recalled that his teacher had asked how he was getting on and he'd said,

I just want it to end.

By 'it' he had meant exams and coursework and university applications – not his life! Elijah did not want to die; on the contrary, he had a clear plan and was looking forward to his future. He wasn't depressed but he was understandably anxious and somewhat overwhelmed. After verbalising his thoughts with me, Elijah said he felt lighter, as if some of the pressure had been lifted. I had listened and normalised his feelings rather than labelling them as something other than ordinary. Elijah did not need or want therapy. He just needed to be listened to. He was not mentally unwell and he did not need specialist psychological support. I wished him well and we said goodbye.

Jimmy

One arena that is awash with labelling is that of looked after children (LAC), which is a label, and sometimes a misnomer, in itself. Many of the LAC and young people I work with do not feel looked after at all. They are placed out of county, away from every thing and every one that is familiar to them. They are assigned a social worker they usually don't like – it's not always personal, it comes with the territory – who rarely visits them because of the distance. The social worker, in role of corporate parent, is responsible for making decisions about and on behalf of the looked after child, and often seems to do so, from what the young people tell me, without consultation. As one young man said to me,

> They know *about* me, they've read the file, but they don't *know* me.

Jimmy had been looked after for six years. He'd had three social workers and seven placements, five with foster families and two in residential care. As well as the label of LAC he had others including ADHD and ODD. His new social worker, whom he had met once, wrote in her referral that she thought he also had pathological demand avoidance (PDA). PDA is one of those labels that really gets my goat. It isn't recognised as a diagnosis in the UK but is often bandied around in relation to children and young people who won't do as they are told. Fifteen-year-old Jimmy was one of those young people. 'Fuck them!' was what he said to me, in relation to all the professionals who were involved in his life. 'Fuck you!' was what he usually said to them. There were a lot of professionals in Jimmy's life. The first time I met him we made a list – social worker, social work manager, independent reviewing officer, advocate, mentor, tutor, sexual health nurse, residential manager, keyworker, twelve residential care staff on rotating shifts, head teacher, class teacher, behavioural unit manager and four behavioural unit members of staff. There were also four previous fostering adults and the staff at his previous residential home. That amounted to over fifty professionals who had read and contributed to Jimmy's file. I was his first psychotherapist. I told Jimmy that I too, had been sent a file. Not a big file but a referral form and a report. I said I was less interested in what other people had to say about him, that was their story, and much more curious to know what he had to say about himself. This was difficult for Jimmy to comprehend. I wondered what he would like me to know about him. He struggled to answer and said there was nothing *to* know. I tried unsuccessfully to coax him into saying something, anything, about who he was, what he did or did not enjoy perhaps, but he seemed totally stumped. Jimmy presented as emotionally shut off. When I wondered about home, school, friends and family he just shrugged and said it was all fine. When I wondered about 'fine' he said,

I've got everything I need

which really struck me. It felt as if he was saying he didn't need very much at all, or perhaps, more likely, that he had learnt not to expect much. After a while Jimmy turned the tables and asked what I knew already 'from the file'. I get asked this a lot by LAC and the question presents a dilemma. My personal belief is that everyone has a right to see what has been written about him or her and that if information is shared among professionals it should also be shared, in an appropriate way, with the young person themself. Many professionals disagree with me and that can make things tricky. It is important to try to work collaboratively with the system around the young person and to think together about how best to support them. Disagreements and differences of opinion can make this difficult. The updated law supports the rights of the individual and states they have the right to access their personal information, and that applies to children and young people as well as adults. What matters in making decisions about whether to share information *about* the child *with* the child is whether they have the capacity to understand the implications – both of accessing the information and about what they might discover if they do (Data Protection Act, 2018). I told Jimmy that his referral mentioned a number of labels. This was factual and seemed like a good place to start to explore and open up a dialogue with him. He said,

> Yeah, I've got ADHD and ASD and that other thing...

He couldn't remember the acronym. I wondered aloud what these labels meant to Jimmy. He said they meant he took medication. I wondered if he thought they accurately described him and he told me he didn't know what they meant. It felt like hard work, as if everything I was curious about was met with resistance. But as I got to know Jimmy I started to realise he wasn't displaying resistance as such, but rather he was illustrating that being thought about was so alien to him that he genuinely had no idea how to respond.

Jimmy told me he was diagnosed with ADHD around the time he first went into care. He said he was angry and always 'kicking-off'. He was excluded from three primary schools by the time he was in year five. When his fourth foster placement ended he was also diagnosed with ODD and given medication to help him sleep. When Jimmy moved into residential care he was assessed and diagnosed with Autistic Spectrum Condition (ASD). He had never been offered access to therapeutic support. When I first met Jimmy I thought he presented as disinterested and, with hindsight, I think that was in part a reaction to his sense that other people were disinterested in him. He told me he used to play in a football team when he was younger and also that he used to go to a youth club. He said that all he did now was play on games consoles in his room because he 'can't be arsed'. When I wondered about when Jimmy lost interest in the things he used to enjoy he remembered it being around the time he went into his third foster placement. It was interesting to me that Jimmy received his first diagnosis around the time he went into care and his enthusiasm for hobbies and interests had waned with every ended placement. When I mentioned it, Jimmy was interested too and agreed when I suggested it seemed significant. He said he used to get angry about being moved and usually responded by smashing things up but he didn't have those feelings anymore. I said it was as if Jimmy's feeling response to being abandoned was so overwhelming that he had learnt to switch it off, and by doing so, other emotions, such as pleasure, had been switched off too. He seemed to understand the link and added spontaneously,

I wonder if I do actually have those things.

I admitted that I was wondering about that too.

Bella

The children and young people I meet often define themselves using language more persuasively than a diagnostic label ever could. Like many LAC, Bella did not perceive herself as cared-about or care-able-about and could not comprehend what was being done to her or why. She seemed disconnected – from me, the work and the wider world around her. She was a dainty little girl who seemed fragile and she reminded me of a butterfly. She flitted and fluttered about the therapy room drawing her attention to and then quickly moving away from things that caught her eye. She picked up crayons, reading books, games, toys, ornaments and would exclaim,

This is nice, how much did it cost?

Bella's curiosity about the value of things illustrated, I think, something of her curiosity about her own value. It was when I suggested this that she likened herself to a five-pound note. She said that like the old paper note, she had been screwed up and passed around between lots of different 'owners'. As well as describing her lived experience of multiple carers, I think this metaphor also expressed Bella's sense of herself as an owned object with very little value.

Teddy

Teddy had a similar sense of himself as worthless. He had experienced multiple placements when I met him aged twelve. Part way through Teddy's second year in therapy I decorated my therapy room. I had prepared him, and all the other young people I was working with at the time, for the changes by showing them the paint colour and wallpaper sample and by counting down the weeks, in the same way I prepare a young person for a forthcoming break or ending. When Teddy came to his first session after the makeover I was disappointed by what I interpreted as disappointment on his face. When I explored this with Teddy I realised that his expression was actually communicating confusion. When I wondered what Teddy felt about the new room he asked me,

> Why would you go to all that trouble for a bunch of care kids?

My response was,

> Because you are worth the effort and because you deserve to have a nice room.

For Teddy, and many in similar situations, the label of LAC literally seemed to mean 'lacking' or 'worth less' than the other, non-LAC, kids.

Kaden

I encourage young people to explore their experiences and the labels assigned to them in their own ways. This can often result in a profound communication that gives me a much greater sense of what it is like for them to be them. My clinical observations suggest a propensity for labels to self-perpetuate and once a young person has been assigned one, more are likely to follow. When I met fourteen-year-old Kaden he had labels of LAC, ADHD, ODD and ASD and was on waiting lists for further assessment. When I mentioned that this was a lot of labels he spontaneously wrote them out on different coloured post-it notes and stuck them on his face. I commented to Kaden that it was difficult for me to see him now, behind the labels, which he took as an invitation to add more – DUMB, LOSER and WASTE OF SPACE. I wondered aloud what it felt like for Kaden to be covered in labels and hidden behind them. He said that people just saw the labels; they didn't see him and that it suited him that way because he could stay 'under the radar'. LAC children and young people often tell me that they feel *looked at* rather than *looked after*. Jimmy's reference to his file is one example of this and Kaden's labels seemed to be another way of saying,

> They know about me but they don't know me.

I wondered to Kaden if he was sick of being looked at and that being under the radar felt like a more comfortable place for him to be. He said it was. I acknowledged that therapy can feel like being looked at too but I hoped this experience would feel different – that I would look at him in a different way and that I would see something that other people might not have noticed. What I was referring to was something akin to the 'maternal gaze' (Winnicott, 2005). Child development theory supports the idea that the infant's sense of self begins to form through their experience of being looked at by their mother, or other primary caregiver. A good-enough carer provides maternal preoccupation by gazing at their baby and taking and expressing pleasure in what they observe. The maternal gaze has a holding function and is also the precursor to the mother/carer functioning as a mirror. The maternal mirror reflects back the infant's own experiences so that he or she learns to internalise a sense of him or herself as separate and feeling in the presence of a separate and feeling other. During the early months, the mother/carer processes feelings on behalf of the infant and then reflects them back in her gaze and her words. For example, a mother might have a sad face in response to a whinging baby and say something like,

Oh, it's not so nice to have that tummy ache.

Or she might smile at her crying baby and say,

I think someone's hungry. Let's get you some lunch.

This gives the infant the experience of their feelings and needs being noticed and understood, so that they gradually learn to notice and understand their own feeling states. But it is not always like this of course. For a whole gamut of reasons, including poor maternal mental health, neglect and abuse, many infants do not have a good enough experience of being 'held' in this way. What the baby sees in the maternal gaze depends on the mother's capacity to mirror and process the baby's experience. Sometimes they are inconsistent, sometimes they get it wrong, and sometimes they are absent. If the mother/carer is unable to mirror and process their baby's experience over a prolonged period of time, not just now and again, the baby might try to avoid the maternal mirror when it does present itself because it feels confusing and deregulating. Infants with these experiences develop into children who are unable to self-regulate, who misunderstand their feeling states and who are misunderstood by others. They often get assigned labels such as ASD, ADHD, attachment disordered, learning disordered or emotionally dysregulated. I can see why, but the labels are not helping children and young people to catch up on what they missed out on as babies, or to develop into mature, feeling, adults. Therapy can help to redress this. The attuned therapist provides something like the maternal gaze and putting their observations into words – 'that seems like a lot of labels' and 'I wonder how it feels to stay under the radar' – can help the young person to feel noticed and attended to so that in time, they can begin to notice and put words to their own feelings in the presence of another.

I encouraged Kaden to think about his post-it note labels one by one and decide what he would like to do with them. He sat in front of a mirror – I don't mean symbolically, I have an actual mirror in my therapy room – and addressed each one in turn. Firstly he peeled off ASD, tore it in half and threw it in the bin. He did the same with ODD. He said LAC was true but he wished it wasn't and decided to put that one away in his therapy box for another time. DUMB and LOSER were folded up really small and followed LAC into the box. Kaden said he probably did have ADHD but he didn't need to have it stuck on him for everyone to see because he didn't want everyone to know. That label got folded up and put in his pocket, which just left WASTE OF SPACE. Kaden said he could think of plenty of people who deserved that label more than he did and that he'd like to see how they would like it if he stuck it on them. I commented that without the labels, I could see Kaden better and that I was learning more about him than the labels could tell me. He pushed the post-it notes and pens towards me and I wrote out some new ones – FUNNY, THOUGHTFUL, CLEVER, INTERESTING. One by one Kaden stuck them on his chest rather than his face, and left them there when his session ended,

So that everyone can see what I'm like.

It might sound as if I am against labelling per se, which I'm not. I have met numerous children and young people for whom thorough, therapeutic assessment has resulted in a diagnosis that has enabled them to access the support that they needed, ultimately changing their lives for the better. What I am against is labelling in lieu of thinking. Therapy provides an opportunity to explore what lies beneath the label, or the file, in order to get to know and make sense of the child or young person. While behaviours and presenting issues might appear similar, the meaning for each individual is always idiosyncratic and nuanced, even if they do share the same label.

References

Data Protection Act (2018).
Jennings, S. (2011) *Healthy Attachments and Neuro-Dramatic-Play*, Jessica Kingsley Publishers, London.
Winnicott, D. (2005) *Playing and Reality*, Second Edition, Routledge, London.

Chapter 4

Sex

A wise man once said,

> I've never worked with a thirteen-year-old for whom sex hasn't been an issue affecting everything at some level.
>
> (Luxmoore, 2016)

I am inclined to agree, and would even go so far as to say that sex is *the* biggest issue that preoccupies adolescents and pre-adolescents. Luxmoore's book 'Horny and Hormonal' was written as a response to his observations over decades working as a school counsellor. In it he acknowledged sexual frissons between students, feelings that teachers might experience towards pupils and even those that pass between counsellors and their adolescent clients. These acknowledgements are honest and brave. I am a big advocate for honest and brave, never more so than when it comes to thinking and talking with children and young people about sex. Honest and brave communication enables us to avoid idealization, demonization or acting out. Unfortunately, most children and young people do not have much opportunity to join with an adult who is prepared to think and talk with them honestly about sex. Many families feel ill equipped, maybe because of their own education (or lack of), or because of their own cultural, moral or religious beliefs, or because of their own embarrassment or fears. What I am saying here is that most adults avoid talking and thinking about sex with young people, on the whole, because of their own inadequacies, insecurities and biases that have nothing at all to do with the young people themselves. This is counterproductive, of course, because it sets up inadequacies, insecurities and biases about sex in the next generation. Some families think it is the schools' job to educate children and young people about sex, but good sex and relationship education (SRE) is sketchy at best. The headlines would have us believe that SRE is compulsory for all young people in secondary education, but legally the only stuff that schools are obliged to teach relates to reproduction and sexual health under the national curriculum for science (Gov.uk). This is informative, but it's not what most children and young people are preoccupied by.

They want to know about real sex, not scientific, diagrammatic sex – how to give or receive a decent blow job, whether you can get pregnant the first time you have sex, how to get someone to have sex with you, how to say no – I've never seen any of that stuff in text books. Schools can opt out from all but the science of sex and/or parents can withdraw their children if they want to. Once again, choices about what is or isn't communicated to young people about sex sit in the hands of adults. Furthermore, academies and free schools are not required to follow the national curriculum at all and so they have free reign about what they do or do not teach in terms of sex and relationship education; that might be nothing or, like I said already, sketchy at best.

Young people I work with in years six, seven and eight sometimes tell me about their scanty sex education and many are left with more questions than answers. One boy, Joe, told me that after watching a 'cartoon' about a man and a woman who were 'supposedly' having intercourse, there was a question-and-answer session. The twelve-year-old boy asked,

What's the point of an orgasm?

which was met with hysterical laughter from his peers and a red-faced,

You don't need to worry about that

from his teacher. I felt frustrated on his behalf. He had been honest and brave and asked a perfectly valid question. I wondered if he would like me to answer it for him and he nodded. My response included a simple scientific explanation,

Well, in terms of reproduction, the male orgasm shoots sperm into the female's vagina, while the female orgasm helps to squeeze it along to where it needs to go.

As well as the less scientific part,

And it can also feel really pleasurable for the person having it.

This response made sense for Joe and left him better informed, less confused and less humiliated. It also meant he was less likely to search out information for himself by entering his question into an online search engine and coming up with who knows what. I wonder why the teacher had dismissed Joe's question rather than respond honestly.

One of the worries adults seem to have is that teaching children and young people about sex will make them go out and do it prematurely, but the evidence suggests that the opposite is true. Another thing I hear a lot from adults is,

They are too young to know

which seems to be a phrase that is bandied around no matter what the age of the child and no matter what the question they are asking. My standpoint is this: if a child is old enough to ask the question, they are old enough to be provided with an age-appropriate answer. I will often explore with a child where their question has originated, particularly if it really does seem premature for the child's age and stage of development. For example, I was rather taken aback when six-year-old Lucia asked me,

What's a virgin?

I played for time by remarking what an interesting question that was and wondering aloud where she had heard the word. Lucia told me she had heard it in a song and it didn't make sense. Relieved and realising that the song was about the Virgin Mary, I said,

A virgin is someone who hasn't made a baby yet.

The answer was factually accurate enough for a six-year-old and meant that Lucia no longer felt confused about a word she was being expected to sing daily in the run up to Christmas. My answer made sense. After the session I let her mother know about her daughter's question and about the answer I had provided. Mum was relieved and said that Lucia had asked her the same thing but that she hadn't known how to respond. My advice is always to be brave and to respond honestly using language that the child will be able to make sense of according to their age and level of comprehension.

Disclosure

There are some questions though that I do not answer: those that relate to my own sex life and/or sexuality. When these questions arise in therapy, as they frequently do, I respond in the same way as I do when I'm asked to disclose anything about my personal life. I say that we are here to think about the young person, not me. Giving a direct answer, such as 'I'm heterosexual' or 'I'm gay' or 'I've watched porn' (or not), would shut down any opportunity for exploration. I ask the questioner why it matters to them to know about my sex life because often it doesn't really matter at all. The question might be asked out of politeness, because the young person doesn't want to offend me or because they are just curious to know. The important thing is not to allow the emphasis to shift onto me and my needs rather than them and theirs. Displacement could well be the reason for the question too, of course. Encouraging the young person, or their parent or carer for that matter, to think about the motivation for the question is much more important than the question or answer itself as it keeps the focus on them rather than me. I then think with them about their motive and respond to that. For example, if a young person says they are curious about my sexuality I might model curiosity and encourage exploration about how we might ascertain someone's sexuality and why it might matter to know. If a young person is grappling with their own sexuality or has just come out as gay or bisexual themselves this might be important to think about because the really pertinent question might be,

How can I know if someone is gay or bisexual like me?

If the reason for asking about my sex life is powered by a desire to avoid offence, I offer reassurance that I have worked with young people for a very long time and have heard about all kinds of sexualities and sexual practices. I let the young person know that the therapeutic space is a place where they can talk openly and honestly about sex, perhaps the only place, and that they will not be judged or criticised on their sexual beliefs or behaviours. But just because I do not disclose anything about my own sexual beliefs and behaviours, it doesn't mean that they aren't relevant. Another reason that personal therapy and/or supervision is so vital to the work that we do as psychotherapists is so that we remain aware of our own unconscious biases and blind spots. The sexual landscape and language have changed immeasurably over the last thirty years or so and it's imperative that we challenge our own attitudes to sex, sexuality, sexual orientation and gender issues. It might not matter whether a therapist is hetero, homo, pan or a-sexual, has had fifty sexual partners or none, but it does matter whether they are open-minded or obstinate. It also matters if their own views are so unyielding that they would potentially infiltrate the work and shut down any opportunity for exploration. If a young person brings a sexual or gender issue to therapy that the therapist feels uncomfortable with because of their own beliefs then they have a duty of care to say so and to refer the client on, because the struggle would belong to the therapist rather than the client and that's not how good therapy works.

Social media

Another arena that gets some adults fired up about children and young people's ages is social media. All the big sites have age restrictions. For Snapchat, Facebook, Twitter, Tumblr, Instagram, Reddit, Ask.FM, ooVoo and Meet Me the lower age limit is thirteen. For Whatsapp it is sixteen and for Whisper, Vine and Tinder it is seventeen. You need to be eighteen to have an account with YouTube, Kik, Musical.ly and Flickr, which is lowered to thirteen with parental permission. That said, I have never met a young person over ten who does not regularly use Snapchat, Instagram, Whatsapp, Tumblr or YouTube to communicate with friends, meet new ones, stream music and videos and share photos, either of their dinner or of their genitalia. They also use social media sites to view porn, learn about sex, engage in virtual sex and hook up for sex in the real world. Sometimes this is age-appropriate, consensual and experimental sex; sometimes it crosses a line. Sometimes the people that children and young people are having sexual experiences with online are of a similar age to them: children and young people who are exploiting the age restrictions too. Sometimes they are adults over eighteen who are using the sites according to the legitimate age restrictions. The paradox is that the main reasons parents and carers mention for prohibiting young people from accessing social media are fears about sexual grooming. This does happen, of course, but it is rare. What most young people are doing online is what generations before them were doing in the real world; they are experimenting with sex and relationships.

Oscar

One boy I worked with, Oscar, had been sent sexually explicit images from an older girl at school via Whatsapp. Initially he was delighted – what heterosexual eleven-year-old boy wouldn't be? But then the girl began sending provocative messages and the boy felt intimidated and out of his depth. He finally told his dad who threatened to report him to the police because he was only eleven and shouldn't be using Whatsapp. That kind of response doesn't stop Oscar or any other young person from accessing sites they are not legally supposed to be accessing, nor does it teach them about safe, consensual sexual behaviour. What it does teach them is to keep schtum about their sexual experiences because adults are not prepared to listen or help them to make sense of them. Another boy, also eleven, had a similar experience to Oscar. I'm calling him Oscar too because it could be the same boy later on or any other eleven-year-old boy. An older girl sent Oscar photographs of herself semi-naked, pictures of her breasts initially but soon the camera travelled below the waist. Oscar was excited by the photographs but also somewhat intimidated. He told his friend about the photographs and his friend asked to see them. Oscar forwarded the images of the girl on to his friend, who forwarded them on to his friend and so on and so on. Eventually, dozens of year six, seven and eight boys were hauled in front of the headmaster and the police to answer charges of sharing sexual images of children. It need not have come to this if the boys had had an adult they could talk to about safe (and legal) sexual experimentation. This happens a lot. I hear dozens of stories from dozens of boys like Oscar and from the girls who make and share sexually provocative images of themselves. This is what young people do and it has become normalised for them. But it can be dangerous and I am careful not to collude while at the same time providing a space where this and any other sexualised behaviour can be explored.

As with any presentation in therapy, I see my role as maintaining a balance between risk and exploration, which is interesting because that's what young people like Oscar are communicating about their early sexual experimentation too. I am careful not to condemn the behaviour and to acknowledge that it is quite ordinary to be excited by photographs of naked or semi-naked bodies. I also encourage young people to explore their feelings response – excitement or arousal perhaps – as well as their thoughts about their own behaviour and the person sharing the images. I also include some psychoeducation because lots of young people don't realise that they are taking, making, storing and sharing sexual images of a child and that this could get them into a whole heap of trouble.

Pornography

As well as viewing images made and shared among their peer group, young people also look at public domain sexual images online. I have worked with children under eight who have viewed pornography but it is more usual for their interest to be piqued in that direction from about the age of eleven up. I would assert that if a child has reached secondary school age they have viewed porn. Lots of adults do not want to accept this but my experience suggests that it is true. Furthermore, these kinds of interests are not surprising or unusual or new. People have viewed images of naked and semi-naked bodies since time immemorial – cave paintings, oil paintings, the lingerie pages of mail order catalogues, so-called 'girlie' magazines, 'lads mags' and erotica. The thing that scares parents and carers now is not finding pictures of bare breasted women or men with bulging y-fronts under their adolescent's bed, but discovering hardcore pornography on their mobile phone. This happens. A lot. However much parents choose to deny it. When I work with parents and carers they sometimes think I'm trying to shock them. In a way I am, I suppose; I'm certainly trying to jolt them into communicating with their child. It is far easier to have an honest conversation with a young person if the adult comes from the position of 'this child will have viewed pornographic images online' rather than 'this child is naïve and would never do something like that'. Coming from a position of normalising sexual curiosity enables honest and brave exploration. Starting from a position of ignorance or denial does not.

Amos

Simon got in touch with me for advice about his discovery of pornographic images on his son Amos' mobile phone. Simon and his wife Annabel had three children: Georgia, sixteen, Finn, thirteen and Amos, eleven. Annabel worked full time and long hours, while Simon worked from home as a graphic designer and took on the majority of the child care tasks. I wondered how the discovery had come about. Simon told me that the rule at home was that all electronic devices had to be left outside of bedrooms after lights out, which varied slightly between the three children according to their ages. Simon admitted that he checked the boys' phones a few times a week to monitor their online activity. I asked if he had spoken to Amos about what he'd discovered, or to his wife – he said he hadn't because he hadn't known what to say. This is not an uncommon response but it is one that frustrates me, in part because it replicates a veil of secrecy and subterfuge. How can we expect children and young people to be open and honest and not keep secrets from their adult carers if adults model secrecy and dishonesty? Simon had contacted me because he wanted to know if Amos' behaviour 'meant something' and if so, what should be done about it. What he was clearly communicating was that he wanted help to make sense of what he had found, firstly for himself and secondly for Amos. I wondered if Simon could remember what he was like at Amos' age. Like Amos, Simon was the youngest of three siblings. He had two older brothers who he recalled talking about sex a lot, not to him, but to each other. As the youngest, Simon had felt left out of those conversations and like most boys of his age at that time he had sneaked a look at 'Page 3' and top shelf magazines whenever he had the chance. I encouraged Simon to draw on his own early adolescent curiosity as a way to normalise the curiosity being displayed by his son. The difference being, of course, that sexual images are much more readily available and accessible than they were when Simon was a child. He relaxed. The behaviour no longer seemed so extreme and Simon had worked out quite quickly that what Amos' behaviour 'meant' was that his son was growing up and developing an interest in sex, as is ordinary and to be expected from a boy of eleven. Our next task was to think about how Simon could support Amos to think about sex without it feeling shaming or duplicitous. I cautioned that he would need to be honest and brave himself if he was going to engender honesty and bravery in his son.

When I met Simon again a month later, he told me he had acted on my suggestion to spend time with Amos away from the house. A common interest that they shared was cycling and for the last two Saturdays Simon and Amos had gone out together on their bikes, stopping for lunch half way through the ride. This had enabled them to be together in a relaxed environment, which had fostered the opportunity to have a relaxed conversation. Simon acknowledged to Amos that he was enjoying observing him grow up into a young man and that he hoped they would always be able to find time to spend together, doing what they both enjoyed, and continuing to learn about each other. It is really important for young people to know they aren't being thought about as babies anymore, even though, in Amos' case, he would always be the 'baby' of the family. Simon did some thinking aloud with Amos about what adolescence had been like for him. Not a warts and all confessional, but a more ordinary sounding,

> I remember having all kinds of questions about all kinds of stuff and not knowing how to work it out...

which normalised the not-knowing position. Simon acknowledged that things were different for young people now and that they can be bombarded with messages and images and that he could imagine how tempting that must be. Simon's aim was to normalise sexual curiosity but his delivery was a bit clunky. Amos smelt a rat and accused his dad of checking his phone. Simon admitted that he had and that initially he had been shocked by what he saw because he hadn't wanted to admit that Amos was not a little boy anymore. He also admitted that he had asked for help to think about what was going on with someone outside of the family (me) demonstrating that he was fallible and that it was ok to ask for help. Because Simon had had an opportunity to reflect and make sense of his own response, he was able to respond to Amos honestly and bravely, which allowed Amos to be honest and brave too. They were able to have a conversation together about how viewing sexual images can be arousing but also that those kinds of images represent a fantasy rather than real life. Amos opened up to his dad about the conversations he'd had at school about how boys and girls should present themselves and what he thought about naked selfies and photo-shopping and filters and the effect they were having on people's self-esteem. Simon was incredibly relieved to have made sense of what Amos' behaviour 'meant' and I have no doubt that Amos was also relieved to be able to have his dad's support to help him to navigate ordinary adolescent sexuality. What I hope this vignette illustrates is the importance of noticing our own response to a child or young person's behaviour, of working out what is our stuff and what is theirs and of making sense of that and reflecting on it, either alone or with help, before we react. This is second nature for most psychotherapists who will have had years of individual therapy themselves in order to sort through and make sense of their own childhood and adolescent experiences. It is also why clinical supervision is so important, so that we have someone else to help us to make sense of our responses with too.

Talking about sex

Lots of young people bring their online experiences to therapy. As in the examples outlined here, specific social media sites or the Internet in general is not really the issue; this is simply the vehicle of expression for real-life explorations of sex and sexual relationships. Taking away young people's phones, banning them from social media or reporting them to the authorities because they are 'too young' does not help them to make sense of sex and relationships. The therapy room can sometimes be the only safe space for children and young people to think and talk freely about sex. They often perceive me as their only reliable source of information and I am comfortable with that. Some counsellors and psychotherapists tell me that children and young people *never* talk to them about sex. I would argue that the reason for that is because they don't feel comfortable, not because they aren't thinking about it or wanting to talk about it, but because they are picking up an unconscious communication that it's not ok to do so. Often adults project their own uncomfortableness onto young people so that they feel uncomfortable too. When they model comfortable, honest communication, as Simon did, they facilitate that in young people. We should not deny or ignore the significance of sex for children and young people because ignorance is not blissful. I see it as an integral part of my role to listen and be alongside children and young people as they try to make sense of sex, in all its myriad forms. They bring questions about their developing bodies, masturbation, menstruation and pregnancy; how it happens as well as how to avoid it, and musings about gender and sexuality; what they are doing, or would like to be doing and who with. The 'how stuff works' questions are often not only brought by younger children (seven, eight and nine year olds) as might be expected, but they are also brought by mid and late adolescents who are presumed to know it all already. Despite their bluster and bravado, and in some instances their sexual behaviour, lots of the adolescents I work with are actually really confused about sex because they have never had a thoughtful parent or parental figure to think about it with. Pre- and mid-teens

regularly bring issues around first sex, safe sex, risky sex and pornography. Film and television storylines and documentaries can
raise awareness about sex, sexuality, sexual abuse and gender, including transgender and gender reassignment. Once these issues
have been raised and emotions evoked, children and young people
have limited choices about where to take them to be thought about
and made sense of. For some young people, the therapy room is one
of the few choices they do have.

At some point in the early twenty-teens there was a cultural sexual
awakening. Erotic literature, predominantly aimed at women, became big business. Pornography came down from the top shelf and
began to take up rows of shelves in bookshops and supermarkets.
Films featuring bondage, domination and sadomasochism began
to dominate the big screen, while soundtracks from 'bonk-busters',
as well as the inevitable accompanying videos, were streamed on
a loop. Eight, eighteen and eighty-year-olds were all singing songs
about sex and it seemed as if everyone was reading about it, watching it and sharing their own sexual fantasies. What seemed difficult
for many adults to acknowledge during this period of sexual revolu-
tion was that children and adolescents had hopped onto the sexual
bandwagon too. Of course they had! They view pornography and
read erotica as part of their sexual education, and once it had gone
mainstream it was more readily available than ever. Young people
look for people to identify with in the real world, online and in the
media in an effort to make sense of their self and their internal
world. They learn through observation and imitation about how to
behave sexually and relationally and they internalise what they see.

Charlie

Children and young people's experiences become internalised and
I notice them in the therapy room. The way that they relate to me in
session is communicative about their relationship experiences, and
that includes sex. Imagine the child or young person who tells me
their intimate personal history in session one, or invites me to sit
very close to them, or 'accidentally' brushes against me, or displays
a lack of self-consciousness in the way they sit: legs apart, hands on
their groin, whether they are male or female. Children and young
people with these presentations are communicating something
about their sexual and relationship experiences, in reality as well
as fantasy. They are also communicating something about the kind

of relationship they want or expect to have with me, which may or may not feel comfortable. I remember a first session with Charlie, a physically well-developed thirteen-year-old girl. She pulled her chair up very close to mine at the table while we were playing a card game. Whenever Charlie put down a card she rubbed against my arm with her breasts. She invited me to reach for something at the other side of her so that somehow, my arm ended up travelling around the back of her shoulders. It was at this point, with my arm in mid air, that I realised Charlie was setting me up me to embrace her. In order to respect our personal boundaries and keep each other safe I said,

> I'm just going to shuffle my chair this way a bit to give us both some more room.

I did not want to humiliate or embarrass her, but it was important to name and maintain the boundary of safe space. I knew that Charlie was sexually active and I suspected that some of her sexual experiences had been non-consensual. She had not learned how to manage herself in a safe, sexual way. Charlie's behaviour in the therapy room was subtle and manipulative and I hypothesised that it mirrored her own sexual experiences of being manipulated and groomed. If I had chosen to ignore or deny what Charlie was setting up between us I would have denied her a valuable opportunity to make sense of her sexual behaviour and, in time, to modify it. This is one of the ways that I am able to offer a different kind of relational experience to the children and young people I work with; by noticing and making sense of, rather than reacting, to their behaviour in the room.

Aliyah

Often young people bring sexual experiences to therapy that are risky and dangerous, sometimes even illegal. This raises ethical dilemmas but my position is always the same – to make sure that the young person can keep himself or herself safe enough, to listen to their story and to help them to make sense of their experience. If I immediately disclosed the risk, then any opportunity to think and make sense would be lost and the young person would continue their unsafe sexual behaviour 'off radar' and arguably that could increase the risk. Managing risk is a delicate balance and I have to make decisions that feel safe enough for me to hold based on my clinical experience and in consultation with my supervisor and sometimes local safeguarding teams in the police or social care services. These decisions are subjective and are different for different therapists. Such dilemmas have been particularly apparent in my work with young people who are engaged in sugar dating – having sex with men for money or gifts. I have read stories in the mainstream press about sugar daddying. They describe female university students joining dating websites in order to earn money to fund their tuition fees, in return for providing company to men. These stories are so heavily diluted that they bear little resemblance to the ones I have heard about in sessions.

I have met lots of young women and girls who talk to me about sugar daddying and so the one I present here, who I'll call Aliyah, is a composite. Aliyah was sixteen when I was asked to offer an assessment following an overdose of alcohol and pills. She told me she hadn't wanted to die; she'd wanted to 'get off her head'. Aliyah was beautiful. Even when I met her that first time in the A&E department, with vomit on her chest, mascara streaking her cheeks and her hair wet through, I could see that she was a naturally attractive young woman. She also seemed very vulnerable and in her helpless, post-binge state I was put in touch with Aliyah the little girl. I warmed to her and I think she sensed that. A&E was a familiar environment for Aliyah. She had been admitted numerous times barely conscious from an excess of alcohol or drugs or both. She felt judged by the hospital staff and sensed their disapproval of her. They tested her bloods and urine while she slept off the effects of her excess, taking up a valuable space in the busy department. The staff discharged her as quickly as they could, expecting her to be back in a week or so after the next binge, which usually she was. Aliyah accepted my offer of individual therapy. She had never had the opportunity to tell her reality before. No one had been interested. Aliyah came to therapy for one year although her attendance was erratic due to her chaotic lifestyle and I sometimes didn't see her for weeks on end. Whenever she did attend I always let her know that I was pleased she had been able to come and that it was good to see her. This reiterated to Aliyah that her attendance was her choice, that I placed no expectations on her and that I would be available for her when I said I would be.

Aliyah told me she had been aware of sugar daddy websites since the age of thirteen. The websites are legal – they are 'just' dating sites – which girls like Aliyah join by uploading sexually provocative photos and fake dates of birth. I guess the people who manage the websites are not too concerned about the actual ages of the girls, who are referred to as sugar babies, because they know that the younger ones attract big business, so they turn a blind eye. I think that lots of adults turn a blind eye when it comes to young people and sex. Aliyah perceived her age as a meal ticket. She said that having sex with an under-age girl was part of the thrill for lots of men and that the younger girls could earn huge amounts of money because, at some level, the men felt guilty. I pointed out that perhaps they felt guilty because they *were* guilty – sex with a child is illegal. Aliyah just shrugged. I didn't press the issue because I knew she knew this, but I did mention it to show that I had acknowledged it. It is one thing to listen to a young person's story and quite another to collude with it. I wondered aloud about how a girl as young as thirteen could keep herself safe in these situations. Aliyah told me that age was also the girls' best weapon. If one of the men gets carried away then he can be reminded that he is having sex with a minor and be threatened with the police. She said they soon 'calm the fuck down' when you remind them of that. As well as age, the other way the girls could up their earnings was from what they were willing to do. Aliyah said,

> To be clear, if you're thirteen and are willing to be tied up or blindfolded or do anal then you're gonna earn loads.

I think she wanted to shock me. I also think she was testing me to see how I would react. I reminded her that I wanted to help her to think about her experiences and that I would neither condone nor condemn them. I also made our contract regarding confidentiality more explicit by pointing out that what she had talked about was hypothetical rather than specific. I said that those kinds of conversations would remain between us in the room. Aliyah knew where the boundary was in terms of confidentiality and disclosure and this allowed her to use the space in a way that felt safe and containing. For months our explorations remained hypothetical, even though we both knew that at some level Aliyah was describing her own experiences, in reality and fantasy.

Aliyah told me that the girls learned to switch off their emotions while they were having sex with men for money. This was a generalised statement about 'girls' and 'men'. We had been working together for a few months when I wondered if Aliyah could own that feeling for herself. She had been talking about her new boyfriend and how he didn't satisfy her sexually. I wondered aloud whether her emotions were switched on or off when they had sex. I encouraged her to think about how she felt physically as well as emotionally when she and her boyfriend were intimate. Aliyah struggled and said she didn't feel anything. She described the sex with her boyfriend as gentle, not what she was used to, and said it didn't feel 'enough'. She said he stroked her and kissed her, which felt weird. I reiterated how difficult it seemed for Aliyah to be in touch with her feelings during sex, but I also acknowledged that she had said the sex didn't feel enough and that it felt weird. This was a start. I normalised 'weird' by agreeing that anything will feel weird if it is new and not what we are used to, and so that feeling made sense. I was curious about Aliyah's description of sex with her boyfriend as not feeling 'enough' and I asked her to elaborate. She said she kept waiting for him to

Bring out the cuffs or the gags or something

but he didn't. I commented that it sounded as if, for him, sex with Aliyah *was* enough, without any gimmicks. Perhaps he was letting her know that she was enough for him. This was difficult for her to hear, let alone accept, but we were at a stage in the therapy where she was able to think about it with me. For so long, Aliyah's defence had been to not think. Sometimes she had tried to shut down my capacity to think about her by drawing me into a provocative narrative or presenting me with yet another dilemma. But eventually Aliyah was able to engage with the thinking part of herself that had been split off.

Because I had been able to think about depraved, illegal sex with Aliyah, I had enabled her to think about it too, in a way that made sense of her experiences for the first time. If I had turned a blind eye I would have colluded with the non-thinking girls who continue to be exploited. If I had shared disclosures and reported stories of underage sex I would have forfeited a relationship with Aliyah that was safe and trusting and which enabled her to engage. The way to change the unthinkable is to think about it.

Arno

Nine-year-old Arno was like a whirlwind; he rushed in, rushed around and rushed out again at the end of the session, on the rare occasions that he managed to stay that long. He was difficult to contain, often needing to go out of the therapy room to the bathroom or to investigate a noise from outside of the room. He picked things up, flung them around and often told me, 'I'm having this' goading me to coax my things back from him. It was difficult to engage Arno in the to-and-fro of conversation or in the turn taking involved in even the simplest games. Most of his activity in the therapy room was solitary and my role for many weeks was to be alongside him, to observe and try to contain him. Within this chaotic presentation, Arno's sexual behaviour was subtle and it took me a while to notice and then make sense of it. His language was full of sexual expletives – fuck, cock, dick, wanker – that spilled out as an accompaniment to his activities. He seemed unaware and I simply observed. This is different to the way that most adults responded to Arno in the real world. I knew they told him that his language was 'inappropriate' and that he should stop it. I do not perceive swearing as inappropriate in the therapy room. Like everything that is said and done, I think of it as a communication. The fact that I did not censor Arno meant that, although nothing was explicit, he was having a different kind of experience with an adult who responded in a different kind of way to the other adults in his world. After a few weeks, Arno became interested in my box of toys. We played simple games together such as Yahtzee and Snap and Arno's capacity to stay with me, with the game and in the room gradually increased. Meanwhile, his sexual language diminished.

During our games, Arno rubbed his groin. There seemed to me to be a link between his capacity to stay-with and his self-soothing behaviour. I noticed this and was curious but I did not verbalise it. It was important to get it right for Arno in terms what I said, as well as when and how I said it. In a later session, Arno's self-soothing became more purposeful. He put his hand inside his shorts, and moved it up and down while repeating aloud,

Dick, dick, dick, dick.

He sounded a bit like a ticking clock, or perhaps more like a ticking cock. Arno was clearly letting me know that he wanted me to notice what he was doing and that he was ready for me to respond. I acted on his cue and said,

It seems as if you want me to notice what you're doing, Arno

He continued to look me in the eye while continuing to say the word, 'dick'. I wondered aloud if he could tell me about what was happening with other words. He told me to guess. I commented,

> Well, you're saying "dick" and it seems as if you are stroking yourself. I'm guessing that feels nice.

Arno said it did and then, to my surprise, he pulled out a pebble from inside his shorts. Immediately what flashed through my mind were the numerous times that Arno had pretended to take things from my room by mimicking putting them down his pants. I was curious but knew it was unlikely that Arno would talk with me about this, so I decided instead to talk to his parents and I invited them in. What I discovered was that Arno had been engaged in rather unusual sexual behaviour for years. His mother seemed relieved to have been given an opportunity to talk about it, while his dad was somewhat dismissive. I encouraged Arno's parents to think back to when they first became aware of something unusual. His mother realised it was when his younger brother, Ernest was born six years ago, when Arno was three. She noticed that Arno used to stroke himself in the bath and would often place his toys between his legs and squeeze them when he was playing. His father admitted he had noticed that too and told Arno to stop it. I knew from the referral and initial consultation that father had a violent temper and that there had been several times when Arno's parents had separated and got back together. They acknowledged that the time around the birth of their second son was particularly fraught. This additional information helped us to contextualise Arno's behaviour and make sense of it. I think it began as a way to self-soothe during a time that felt traumatic due to the birth of a sibling, parental disharmony and separation. The behaviour became sublimated through fear of his father's recriminations. It did not go away because it served an important purpose, to disavow overwhelming feelings that infant Arno was unable to verbalise, but it did become hidden and habitual. The term 'disaffection' is used to describe an inability to put words to feelings, particularly fitting for individuals who have experienced overwhelming emotion. This fits with my sense of chaotic, uncontained Arno who was a vulnerable boy trying to demonstrate that he was a strong, sexual man, and a good enough match for his father.

The psychoanalyst Joyce McDougall suggested that disaffected individuals have,

> ...an inability to contain and reflect upon an excess of affective experience.
>
> (McDougall, 1989)

It is therefore the job of the parent and/or therapist to contain and reflect on their behalf until such a time that their capacity increases. I encouraged Arno's parents to verbalise their observations of Arno's sexual behaviour rather than judge, punish or ignore it. They practiced some simple phrases such as, 'it seems you have put something inside your pants' or 'I've noticed you are rubbing your penis' and to add something to show that they understood Arno's motivation such as, 'maybe that feels nice'. Gradually the behaviour diminished, as Arno began to feel less overwhelmed by his feelings and more contained by his parents.

So far, in this chapter about sex, I have included vignettes of my work with three children aged six, nine and thirteen. Some readers will not have noticed their ages until now, while others will have been shocked by my discussion of the sexual lives of children. My clinical experience supports the notion that the origins of sexual urges, behaviours and desires, which Freud collectively termed 'libido' can be traced back to infancy (Freud, 1896), where tensions are set up between primitive internal drives to comfort, soothe and satisfy, and external cues that disallow them. My work with Arno's parents focused on exploring the significance of their son's masturbatory behaviour and his choice of sexual objects and it did not surprise me to learn that his behaviour could be traced back to early childhood origins. If we think about libido more generally as any kind of physical pleasure, rather than specifically sexual gratification, it is perhaps not such a leap to accept that the behaviour that infants rely on for comfort throughout infancy and childhood are the same behaviours that drive their sexual desires into adolescence.

Eamon

My clinical experience supports the notion that,

> ...human sexuality is inherently traumatic
>
> (McDougall, 1996)

particularly for young people struggling to make sense of their sexual preferences. Seventeen-year-old Eamon asked his mother to find him a therapist to manage issues, according to the referral, relating to social anxiety. I met them together for an initial consultation. Eamon was a tall, well-built young man, attractive and a bit awkward looking, as if he was not quite comfortable in his own skin. His mother was supportive of Eamon's request for therapy and explained that he had always been shy and self-conscious, even as young boy. This was illustrated in the here-and-now by his propensity to blush and perspire. Eamon's body betrayed any attempts he made to disguise his feelings. He wafted his hands around in front of his face and tugged at the neck of his shirt. I commented that he seemed to be 'hot under the collar' and suggested we slow down and take things at a gentler pace. Eamon was happy to let his mother do most of the talking during the consultation but was also keen to arrange individual sessions. There seemed to be some urgency in his request and I had a sense that he was very certain what he wanted to work on.

During Eamon's initial individual sessions, he told me within the first moments that he had 'a problem with intimacy' and was unable to maintain an erection. He blurted this statement out as if it was a confession he needed to get rid of. He blushed and started to perspire, as he had in the consultation, and then he sobbed uncontrollably. Suddenly, I was no longer in the room with a young adult male, but instead I was in the presence of a desolate little boy. I held in mind these two parts of Eamon, the sexual man and the vulnerable child. I acknowledged that, for reasons I did not yet understand, Eamon had separated parts of his psychological self as a defence against an overload of unbearable, overwhelming feelings. The psychoanalyst Melanie Klein referred to this kind of splitting of the self as 'fragmentation'. She saw it as an ordinary and necessary part of healthy maturation and a feature of the paranoid-schizoid state of mind (Segal, 1988). According to Klein, paranoid anxieties and schizoid defences are gradually relinquished, but fragmentation can be a feature of regression and illustrates a defensive form of psychological functioning. I could not yet know what Eamon was defending himself against but there were strong unconscious communications; my sense that he seemed uncomfortable in his own skin/body, that his physiological responses of blushing and perspiring betrayed any attempt to hide his underlying feelings and his tendency to get embarrassed and 'hot under the collar'. I also

wondered about the possible symbolism of Eamon's early disclosure of erectile dysfunction, which could be considered premature
or perhaps precocious.

Over a period of months, we explored Eamon's difficulties in the
context of his relational experiences and we gradually made sense
of them. He had experimented sexually with girls during his early
teens and lost his virginity aged fourteen-and-a-half with an older
girl aged seventeen. The experience had not been satisfactory. The
girl was a friend of a friend he had hooked up with at a party. She
was nice, they had flirted and kissed, and Eamon was 'desperate'
to get 'it' – first intercourse – out of the way, so they had sex. I acknowledged aloud that it sounded as if his virginity felt like something he wanted to get rid of urgently, like his disclosure to me in
the first moments of the first session that had seemed premature
and precocious. Eamon said that the second his erect penis went
anywhere near the girl it went limp leaving him feeling inadequate
and ashamed. I wondered if he had any idea why having sex had felt
so urgent; he had only been fourteen-and-a-half after all. Eamon
said he wanted to be like the other kids, by which he meant the
other boys. He described them as full of bravado about what they
fantasised doing with girls and boasts about what they apparently
had. Eamon then finally said aloud for the first time that he was
gay. His acknowledgement made sense of my observations; the way
his body betrayed any attempts to hide his feelings; by blushing,
sweating, crying and dysfunctioning, and the sense I had that he
was uncomfortable in his own skin.

Eamon told me that in the last six months before accessing therapy he had started meeting up with men he met online. Inevitably,
the men wanted sex, which Eamon declined because he was fearful
about anal penetration and still unsure about what would satisfy
him sexually. A couple of times he had masturbated the men he
dated but he had never experienced an erection, either with them
or when he masturbated alone. And so the sense of dissatisfaction
and inadequacy continued. Things changed when Eamon met Rav
who was able to arouse him by pinching his abdomen and but-
tocks really hard to the point that it left marks on his skin. This felt
double-edged for Eamon; he was finally able to enjoy sexual satis-
faction, yet in a way that seemed (to him) abnormal. What struck
me was both that Eamon had subverted pleasure and pain, and also
that his sexual gratification was assigned to non-genital parts of his
body, which is sometimes referred to as partialism. Although the

behaviour was non-penetrative, Eamon experienced it as sexually arousing. It enabled him to achieve and maintain an erection and he referred to it as sex. Eamon described sex with Rav as an almost hallucinatory experience. He also questioned whether it was a perverse kind of fetish. In Theatre of the Mind, Joyce McDougall (1982) writes that,

> The perverse sexual act functions like a dream, a kind of hallucinatory creation of an alternative reality and serves as a solution to avoid painful internal conflicts.

I think McDougall uses the term 'perverse' to mean unusual rather than abhorrent. I knew from my explorations with Eamon of his early sexual experiences that his internal conflict centred on his need to repress his sexuality. He had engaged in disingenuous and dysfunctional heterosexual activity followed by a tentative and dysfunctional exploration of homosexuality. It made sense that he had (unconsciously) redirected any sexual pleasure away from the genital area, which he associated with sexual dysfunction and shame. Once this was understood, Eamon was less self-critical, more at ease with himself and more ready to expand his repertoire of sexual behaviours.

Very few children and young people present their sexual behaviours with an explicit wish to change them. They often share premature sexual experiences and we cannot turn back the clock. Many of the young people I listen to are embarrassed, ashamed or confused about their sexual experiences. In part this is because of their internal sense of self, but also, often, it is because of how their sexual behaviour has been judged by adults as something to be embarrassed or ashamed about. I have heard stories about sex that are shocking, some that are disgusting and others that are illegal. I always keep in mind the safety of the child or young person in the here-and-now and I check in regularly to make sure that they can keep themselves safe enough. With one eye on risk, I can turn the other to exploring the young person's narrative through a psychodynamic lens. I share as much or as little of my thoughts and interpretations as I think they might find helpful. What is most reassuring for most children and young people to hear is that, thought about in context, their sexual behaviour makes sense. This frees them up to make sense of it too and to accept it, change it or let it go.

References

Freud, S. (1896) *The Aetiology of Hysteria*, Standard Edition Volume 3, Vintage, London.

Luxmoore, N. (2016) *Horny and Hormonal*, Jessica Kingsley Publishers, London.

McDougall, J. (1982) *Theatre of the Mind: Illusion and Truth on the Psychoanalytical Stage*, Free Association Books, London.

McDougall, J. (1989) *Theatre of the Body: A Psychoanalytic Approach to Psychosomatic Illness*, Free Association Books, London.

McDougall, J. (1996) *The Many Faces of Eros*, Free Association Books, London.

Segal, H. (1988) *Introduction to the Work of Melanie Klein*, Karnac Books, London.

Statutory Guidance on Sex and Relationship Education. www.gov.uk/government/publications/sex-and-relationship-education. Last updated 25 July 2019 (accessed 22 August 2019).

Chapter 5

Identity

Children and young people develop in stages. Their development is linked to physiological changes and those associated with chronological age, but it is not necessarily linear and it concerns areas way beyond the realms of biology. As well as physical growth, social, intellectual, emotional and psychological development all contribute to a person's sense of who they are, or what we might more commonly refer to as identity. So too, the family environment as well as the wider social and cultural context impact a child and young person's sense of self in relation to other people in their own world and the wider world at large. The initial stage of development happens in utero. It can be difficult to fathom how the experience of the developing foetus might be related to the identity of an adolescent, but evidence and clinical experience supports that it is. That is one of the reasons why, when I meet a child or young person who has been referred to therapy, whatever their age or stage of development, I start with an initial consultation which includes an exploration of development starting with conception, pregnancy and birth. Childhood denotes the stage of development from birth to puberty, which is marked by a multitude of developmental milestones: feeding and weaning, talking and walking, separation and loss and countless transitions along the way. Puberty marks the beginning of adolescence, which is the transitional stage between childhood and adulthood. Every single experience, milestone and transition, from conception onwards, contributes to the development of identity. In addition, the different perceptions of those experiences and transitions, from parents and carers, as well as the perception of experience of child themself will influence their developing identity. A full theoretical exploration of child development is beyond the scope of this text, but it is worth focusing on one particular stage of development that is so often fraught with friction, tension and confusion around identity, and which so often results in referrals to psychotherapy – that of adolescence. Adolescence, like any stage of maturation, has its own set of developmental tasks. These include separation from family, integration of self and development of identity.

Eros and Thanatos

I like the definition of adolescence as a period of 'sturm und drang' (Hall, 1904), which has a literal translation of storm and stress. This sums up the experience of most adolescents quite nicely. The pressure (stress) to achieve – academic success, financial and emotional independence, popularity, sexual prowess – is rife, at a time when storming hormones are changing young people's bodies both inside and out. Instability and turmoil come with the territory, even for adolescents growing up within a stable, loving family, while those living in an environment furnished with chaos and violence are likely to present as chaotic and violent themselves and/or as emotionally shut-off and socially isolated. Adolescents are often labelled as 'hysterical'. The term is used to describe their feverish, excited emotional reactions, or their behaviour, which can be manic or distraught. I often hear about adolescent responses that seem more exaggerated or extreme than the situation warrants. The teen who absconds or cuts themselves in response to a low test score or an argument with a friend, for example. When Freud wrote about hysteria in the late nineteenth century, he asserted that,

> In so far as one can speak of determining causes which lead to neuroses, their aetiology is to be looked for in sexual factors.
>
> (Freud, 1895)

As this quote illustrates, Freud, not surprisingly, made a link between hysteria and sex. One of the key features of psychotherapy is the transference, and I have mentioned this briefly elsewhere. Transference is a psychodynamic concept that can be difficult to comprehend. It is the phenomenon whereby a client unconsciously transfers feelings originating from a situation in the past onto the therapist in the here and now. So, for example, a young woman might treat her therapist with disregard or contempt, due to the relationship she has with her mother. We might think of this as maternal transference, because the client relates to the therapist, in the transference, *as if she were her mother*. Sometimes the transference relationship is subtle, at other times it is difficult to ignore. For example, I've lost count of the number of times a child or young person I'm working with has called me by another person's name; the person they were unconsciously relating to me as, as if I were that person.

Countertransference, then, is the therapists' unconscious feelings towards their client, which can come about as a result of, or lead to over-identification. To take the same example of the client with the difficult mother/daughter relationship, if I am working with that client and she treats me with contempt, *as if I were her mother*, and if I have a daughter or son of a similar age, I might react as if I were the client's mother, with a retaliatory comment or a rebuff. This would not be helpful, of course, which is why it is vital to attend to, process and make sense of any and all countertransference feelings, either during personal reflection and/or in supervision. Transference and countertransference responses provide valuable information about the therapeutic relationship in the here and now, as well as the client's past and current relationships. What happens in the transference can also be informative about the child or young person's sense of self: their identity in relationship with another.

When working with adolescents, because so much of their preoccupation is to do with sex, we might find ourselves caught up in, what is known as, erotic or sexualised transference. This relates to transference in which the clients' fantasies about their therapist are romantic or sexual in nature. There are professionals working with children and young people who deny the existence of erotic transference in their work, arguing that it only relates to adult therapy. My response to that is balderdash! As with any denial of or splitting off of feelings, I think this is a hazardous position to take because it sends the feelings underground. Children and young people are sexual beings with sexual and sensual feelings and fantasies. It makes sense that some of those feelings and fantasies would be directed towards their therapist with whom they share a close personal relationship. Erotic transference can manifest as flattery, flirtation, innuendo or outright invitation. I have experienced a whole gamut of so-called 'erotic' experiences in therapeutic sessions: the girl who talks to my breasts rather than my face, the boy who repeatedly draws penises, the one who masturbates, the adolescent who wonders if I like 'fucking'. Situations like these can be daunting, for inexperienced as well as more seasoned professionals. The key, as always, is to maintain safe boundaries, assess risk and make sense of what's going on in the room, consciously and unconsciously. The same is true in instances of erotic countertransference; intimate or sexual feelings the therapist may experience towards their client. These can arise as a result of being pulled into the erotic transference, or for other reasons. It is imperative to acknowledge the feelings and to make sense of where they have originated and what they might be about.

Nothing is certain for adolescents and very little will stay the same as it used to be. No wonder then that they are likely to present as isolated and shut off one minute, fiery and argumentative the next. The mood and behaviour of adolescents seems unpredictable because it is both a reaction to and a projection of the unpredictable stage of development they are experiencing, and will continue to experience for fifteen years or more. Yes, that's right; fifteen years! The developmental stage of adolescence stretches from puberty to mid-twenties.

Children are displaying signs of physical development younger than ever before. Onset of puberty has decreased, for girls in particular, with many showing first signs of sexual development at eight. Numerous theories have been posited for this including diverse factors such as nutrition, pollution, the absence or presence of fathers, increased affluence and over-exposure to television (BBC News, 2015). The long, slow transition from childhood to adulthood also stimulates psychological consideration about life, the universe and everything. Many adolescents become contemplative or philosophical, and develop an interest in psychology, philosophy, politics and existential debate. What they are trying to work out is who they are and where they fit in this great big world. Other (or the same) adolescents develop interests in drugs and alcohol and other risky and potentially life threatening activities including self-harm and suicidal ideation. All of adolescent behaviour, the contemplative *and* the risky, is both ordinary and terrifying. And all of it, when it is broken down to its basic origins, is about sex and death.

Freud was the first to identify an enduring conflict between life and death. He referred to the sexual and self-satisfying life instinct, Eros, and the antagonistic and hostile death instinct, Thanatos (Freud, 1930). In my view, Eros and Thanatos symbolise adolescence personified. For adolescents, absolutely everything is perceived as a matter of life or death. Academic underachievement (or perceived underachievement), friendship, family and other relationship break-ups, not being allowed to stay out late or go to the party that 'everyone' is going to or have the trainers or jacket or games console that 'everyone' has can feel like the end of the world for an adolescent, or more accurately, the end of *their* world. Ditto confiscation of their phone, a declining number of 'followers' on social media or a low number of 'likes' on their post. The list really is endless. The reason that these experiences feel so unbearable for adolescents is because they threaten their sense of self at a time when it already feels so fragile. Not being at the party or not having the trainers or not maintaining a popular enough and like-able enough social media profile threatens the adolescent's identity at a time when it is not yet robust enough to withstand such attacks. This is true of ordinary adolescents developing in an ordinary way in an ordinary enough family. Throw an additional unexpected or unwelcome variable into the mix – say loss, illness, neglect or any kind of abuse – and the effects can be experienced as catastrophic.

Initial episodes of self-harm, or first thoughts about suicide, are often triggered during adolescence by experiences such as these, which challenge the young person's sense of identity. So, when an adolescent presents with suicidal ideation it does not necessarily mean that they intend to end their life or have the motivation to do so and thankfully, occasions when that happens are extremely rare. What it does mean is that they are contemplating their own life and mortality and we should take their communication seriously – not dismiss it as a silly over-reaction, nor over-react ourselves and become hypervigilant and cosseting. I do a lot of thinking, with adolescents in particular, about life and death. This can help to identify the internal alive and internal dead parts of their self, which leads in theoretical terms to resolution of the life/death conflict. The adolescent who has their fears, fantasies and feelings about death taken seriously becomes less fragmented, their desire to deaden parts of their self diminishes and they are freed-up to continue the journey into adulthood with alive, sexual potential, which of course is what it's all about. The potential for sex is a major preoccupation for the majority of adolescents raising questions such as – Who am I? Who am I attracted to? Who is attracted to me? Who will I have sex with, when, how, where and how often?

Harry

A question that is often asked of and by adolescents is 'how do you identify?' I cannot recall when this became common parlance but it was relatively recently and certainly within the last decade. The question relates specifically to gender and sexual identity, which can be linked but are also distinguishable. I met a mother, Carol, and her sixteen-year-old son, Harry, for an initial consultation. Carol described her son as 'obsessed' by gender and sexuality as if it had become a 'hobby' for him. She said that he identified his peers, not by name or appearance, but in terms of 'my gay friend' and 'the bisexual one' or 'the one who is pan'. Carol was baffled. The family had sought my help to address (what they referred to as) Harry's 'excessive sexual behaviour'. Following an initial introduction of 'the issues' as perceived by Carol, we spent some time reflecting on her relationship with Harry's father and the pregnancy that resulted in the birth of their son. Carol met Andy when she was thirty-eight and he was fifty-two. He was her married boss and their relationship was brief, passionate and tumultuous. The pregnancy was unplanned and Andy made it clear that, while he would provide financial support, he had no desire to be involved in the upbringing of his illegitimate child. Carol's pregnancy resulted in Andy's separation from his wife to whom he had four other sons who were already in late adolescence and early adulthood at the time that Harry was born. Carol and Andy attempted to live together for a short time during baby Harry's first year, but their relationship did not stand the test of ordinary, mundane, day-to-day life and they separated within six months. Andy came in and out of their life during Harry's childhood. There were numerous attempts at reconciliation that came to nothing, followed by periods of absence for months and sometimes years. I commented that the parental relationships sounded complicated and perhaps at times confusing for everyone concerned. I was struck by the themes of forbidden and passionate sex, the unplanned consequences of the extra marital affair, and the numerous break-ups and make-ups. The narrative that had been presented of Harry's childhood was one of inconsistency and it involved a lot of sex. I thought it sounded very adolescent and there was little wonder then that sex was the presenting issue in the here and now for adolescent Harry.

When I asked Harry if he was in a relationship, he told me,

I've been seeing one or two people.

I hear lots of adults talking the way that Carol did, professionals as well as parents and carers, whose views and vocabulary are so alien to young people. I invited Harry to say what it was like for him that his mother had the views that she did about sexuality. He said it made it impossible for him to talk to her, which he would really like to be able to do.

I see my role, in part, as helping to facilitate communication between parents and their children. In an ideal world no young person would need to visit a psychotherapist or counsellor because they would be able to talk openly to their parent or carer about whatever it was that happened to be troubling them. Their parent or carer in turn would be able to listen and help them to make sense of it. Lots of parents say to their sons and daughters something like 'you can talk to me about anything' but what they actually hear when their children do talk to them will always be coloured by their own views, experiences and prejudices, as well as by their emotional connection to their child. In consultation with Carol and Harry I did some thinking aloud, as I often do. I said that I had been noticing the different language they each used to talk about sexuality. Carol did not name it. She described the boys at school as 'not normal' and 'the other way'. While for Harry, sexuality and the language he used to describe it was ordinary, comfortable and explicit. I commented on Carol's description of Harry as 'obsessed' by gender and sexuality and acknowledged that I could see why she might think that. I said that for lots of young people like Harry, who are working out who they are and whom they are attracted to; sex and sexuality can become something of a preoccupation. I also stated that this is a quite ordinary and important task of adolescence. I agreed too that it could seem as if sex was a 'hobby' for adolescents while they are busy experimenting with their thoughts, feelings and behaviours. My aim was to let Carol know that I had acknowledged and validated her concerns and confusion while also normalising Harry's thoughts and behaviours as part of ordinary adolescence and the ordinary adolescent task of identity development.

Gender

As the consultation with Carol and Harry illustrates, the way that young people think and talk about sexuality is often poles apart from their parents' or carers' perceptions and vocabulary. Many adults can recall a time when homosexuality was illegal – it was decriminalised in England and Wales in 1967, in Scotland in 1981 and remained illegal in Northern Ireland until 1982. The age of homosexual consent was only lowered to sixteen in 2001. The acronym LGB only entered common parlance during the 1980s and at first included just lesbian, gay and bisexual. Today, it is broadly accepted that sexuality cannot be reduced to homosexual or heterosexual and so too the concept of gender is less likely to be defined in binary terms. In the 1990s the acronym LGB was extended to include T for transgender and then Q, which can stand for queer or questioning, and + to include any and all other sexual or gender identities. That was almost thirty years ago and so what that means is that the language denoting sexual and gender identity that adults find so confusing is just ordinary and everyday to children and young people because it has always existed in their lifetime. The 'new' vocabulary recognises difference and brings with it a level of acceptance.

On the whole, most children and adolescents are more accepting of gender and sexual difference than most adults, but they still need help to make sense of it. Choice, fluidity and acceptance bring their own set of difficulties. When the socially accepted norm was for boys to be boys who were attracted to and had sex with girls, and for girls to be girls who were attracted to and had sex with boys, people knew what was expected of them and acceptable by society. Choice can be confusing. Carol talked about the 'seeds' that are planted in children's minds by formal sex education in school and self-education via the Internet. In a way she is right – children *are* presented with a range of ideas and options that adults were not when we were adolescents, but I don't think this is what persuades them to 'jump on the bandwagon'. I think instead that it gives young people permission to explore their sexual and gender identity and a language with which to express it. It also lets them know that they do not have to fit into a pigeonhole or be defined by a narrow stereotype or expectation of what gender and sexuality mean. This is helpful because it is accepting and non-discriminatory, but it is also challenging because the spectrum is so vast.

What is sometimes referred to as gender variance is a relatively recent visitor to the therapy room. According to the Tavistock and Portman, there has been a doubling of referrals to their specialist Gender Identity Development Service, which offers support to gender variant and transgender children and young people under the age of eighteen (Gender Identity Development Service, 2016). In the wider population, it is estimated that approximately

0.005–0.014 percent of individuals who are assigned male at birth are later diagnosed with gender dysphoria. The figure for those who are assigned female at birth is between 0.002 and 0.003 percent. These figures are based on the number of people who seek formal support from specialist services and so the actual prevalence of gender dysphoria is likely to be much higher (DSM-V, 2013). The charity Barnardos offers specialist support to children and young people with a wide range of complex issues. They also have a specialist Positive Identities service that offers training to professionals with the aim of raising awareness of LGBTQ issues, promoting inclusion and tackling homophobic, biphobic and transphobic bullying. Barnardos suggest that as many as two percent of the population are gender variant or transgender; which, to put that figure into perspective, is the same percentage of people who have red hair. Many adults are struggling to comprehend the concepts of gender fluidity, gender questioning, gender variant and transgender. I have met numerous adolescents for whom therapy is a way to make sense of their developing gender identity and in each case we have explored what it means to them in the context of their family and developmental background: no assumptions, no prejudices, and absolutely no preconceived ideas.

Nicky

Nicky was born female and came to therapy to explore her feelings of wanting to be a boy. Nicky dressed in boy's clothes and shoes, had a short, boyish haircut and never wore makeup. She preferred to hang out with boys and was interested in traditionally boyish activities such as skateboarding and mountain biking. Her family thought of her as a tomboy. Her mother accepted Nicky's preferences but perceived them as a phase she would grow out of. There was possibly some truth in that perception. The majority of children and young people who question their gender do not continue to do so following puberty (NHS, 2019). Nicky's father was less accepting. He did not understand it, refused to talk about it and did not engage in the therapeutic process. You may have noticed the language and pronouns I have used in relation to Nicky. I have stated that she dressed in boys' clothes, had a boyish haircut, was interested in boyish activities and conveyed feelings of wanting to be boy. This was the language expressed by the family in our initial consultation. I am always careful to use the vocabulary that is presented to me rather than my own, so that I present the family's narrative rather than mine. That said, I do sometimes challenge the use of language, often with the aid of humour as I did with Nicky and her mother when I asked the rhetorical question,

Who says that girls can't ride skateboards or have short hair?

They smiled and it relieved some of the tension.

What I learnt about Nicky, from listening to her over a number of individual psychotherapy sessions, was that she did not identify with the traditional concept of what it means to be a girl and that she did not feel as if she had much in common with the girls at school. As a consequence, she had experimented with what it might be like to be a boy. We tried to explore when she was first aware of her sense of difference. Nicky had experienced an early puberty. She started her periods at nine and wore her first bra soon after. This was much earlier than her friends and it made her feel uncomfortable about her body from about school Year 5 She remembered feeling envious of the boys who 'didn't need to think about that stuff' and continued to play, unencumbered by things as inconvenient as breasts and menstruation. Most of the girls did too at that age but Nicky knew what they had coming. The more she thought about the differences between girls and boys, the more she felt she identified with the latter. By the time she started secondary school, Nicky was choosing all her clothes from the boy's rails in shops, had cut her hair short and had been flattening her breasts with sports bras and layers of lycra to disguise her feminine curves. Her outward presentation was masculine but her preferred pronouns were 'she' and 'her'. Nicky told me she didn't identify as male or female and I suggested that she seemed to sway between the two. She agreed and seemed relieved that she didn't have to fit herself into a gender box that didn't suit her, at least not in the therapy room.

I wondered why she felt she had to be certain about her gender out there in the world. She said that she had spoken to a teacher, well meaning enough, who had suggested to her that she might have gender dysphoria. This diagnosis is used when a person's gender identity is contrary to the gender assigned at birth, so when a person born female identifies as male or vice versa. Gender dysphoria has replaced the previously used diagnostic label of gender identity disorder (DSM-V, 2013), and in doing so dis-ease has been replaced with un-ease, which is less stigmatising and more accepting, rather like the extended acronym LGBTQ+. But gender dysphoria is still

I wondered if they were male or female and he said 'both'. It didn't matter to me whether Harry identified as heterosexual, homosexual, bisexual or something else, but I wanted to illustrate with my question that I was making no assumptions. Carol rolled her eyes, both at my question and at her son's answer. The way we think and talk about sexual orientation has changed. Until relatively recently we were conditioned to accept, at least publicly, the social norm of heterosexuality and to think of gender in binary terms. Many people – parents, carers and professionals – remain fixed to that heterosexist/binary notion and Carol seemed to be one of them. Some psychologists, on the other hand, have suggested that sex and gender should be conceptualised, not as switches that point this way or that, but rather as a series of adjustable dials. Within this framework, neither sex nor gender are either/ors but instead are continuous spectrums. These theoretical dials influence hormone levels and development in utero and at puberty, as well as personality traits, and social, historical and cultural factors (Pirlott and Schmitt, 2014). The dials not switches model supports the view that gender identity is less likely to be entirely male or entirely female and more likely to be something in between, perhaps something more akin to gender fluidity, and that sexuality too is less likely to be binary, no matter how we identify. Young people seem to 'get' this and accept it as their norm. Many adults, on the other hand, struggle to comprehend.

I let Carol know that I had noticed her roll her eyes and I wondered if she could explain what it was like to hear her son admit that he had relationships with peers who were both male and female. She told me she didn't understand it. She said,

> When I was at school there were a couple of boys who, looking back, I could see were not normal. I know now that at least one of them turned out to be the other way.

She said she was ok with that, so long as they didn't 'rub it in your face' but that it was different now... She trailed off and I wondered if she could say how she thought things were different today to when she was at school in the late 1970s and early 1980s. She said,

> Well these days, the school and the Internet plant seeds in children's minds and then they jump on the bandwagon saying they are this or that one minute, then change their mind the next.

a label, with all the trappings that labels bring, and it is often used, as in Nicky's case, inappropriately. Nicky was an ordinary adolescent, grappling with ordinary adolescent questions about her identity, including gender identity. She was acutely aware of her developing body and that it was changing faster than she was comfortable with. In fact everything was changing faster than she was comfortable with: school, friends, social politics, the climate.... She said it was hard for her to keep up! Once the pressure to confirm to a specific gender was alleviated, Nicky was freed up to think with me about other ordinary adolescent stuff and admit how confusing it all was. And once all of the ordinary, confusing stuff had been normalised, Nicky was soon thinking about it with her parents as well, who had the difficult challenge of adapting to the role of parents-to-an-adolescent rather than parents-to-a-little-girl, which is ordinary and confusing too.

Ayesha

Ayesha was assigned biologically male at birth and identified as trans-female. She had a diagnosis of gender dysphoria from a specialist gender identity service. I called Ayesha by her preferred name and referred to her using her preferred pronouns, 'she' and 'her'. This was not awkward it was reality. Ayesha was seventeen-and-a-half when I met her and she had already encountered numerous professionals including psychologists, psychiatrists, psychotherapists and counsellors. She felt let down by them all. It felt to Ayesha as if every time she met someone new that before long they dropped her. Some supported her for a while and then left the service they worked for. Some met her a few times and then referred her on to colleagues because their caseload was too big, and another had referred her on because of her age. Ayesha had not felt as if anyone 'got it'. She told me about the psychologists who asked too many questions and the psychotherapists who sat in silence with straight faces not really engaging. I found that observation particularly interesting. I get lots of referrals about children and young people who are described as 'not engaging' with previous professionals. No one ever says anything about previous professionals not engaging with *them*! Any kind of counselling or psychotherapy – or tutoring or teaching or parenting or caring for that matter – is a two-way street and we need to be ready and willing to engage *with each other* if the relationship is going to work. The level of reality in

Ayesha's accounts of the professionals she had met before me was neither here nor there. What was important was what she was communicating about the kind of relationship she needed from me – one where she felt supported and held rather than rejected and one where she felt understood and responded to on a relational level. I shared my thoughts about this with Ayesha and she agreed that I had hit the nail on the head.

The reason that Ayesha was presenting in therapy (again) was because she wanted help to navigate the dilemmas of transitioning. Despite some people's misconceptions (at best) and scare mongering (at worst), the vast majority of treatments available to individuals diagnosed with gender dysphoria are psychological rather than physiological; that's why, like Ayesha, they meet so many professionals with the prefix 'psych'. It is understood that family and early developmental experiences are significant contributing factors to adult gender identity, (Gender Identity Development Service, 2016). Therefore, an important component of the psychological support offered to young people includes an exploration of family relationships and early developmental history – which I advocate as part of any psychotherapeutic intervention no matter what the presenting issue. In other words, therapeutic interventions for children and young people presenting with gender variance, dysphoria or confusion aim to assess, explore, support, reflect and make sense of their experiences from birth onwards, just like any other therapeutic intervention.

That said, medical treatments are sometimes offered and they can be hugely beneficial. Most children with a diagnosis of gender dysphoria experience puberty as overwhelming as their body becomes more like their assigned gender and less like their gender identity. In these instances, synthetic hormone treatment may be prescribed to reduce the physiological changes associated with pubertal development. Ayesha experienced puberty as excruciating. She had already presented in her preferred gender identity at home and school for a number of years when the inevitable pubertal changes started to become apparent. She was repulsed by her enlarged penis, muscle development and male pattern hair growth. She started shaving every accessible part of her body at the age of nine and this soon morphed into harming herself by cutting the body she despised with a razor almost daily. From the age of ten she tucked and taped her penis every morning meaning that she didn't go to the toilet during the school day because it was almost physically impossible. She developed urinary tract infections and cystitis, stomach pains and bloating. She learnt to control her bladder by not drinking anything all day and she became weak and dehydrated. But all that physical discomfort was preferable to being faced with the reality of her biological body.

Ayesha started taking gonadotrophin-releasing hormone analogues when she was thirteen, after suffering physically and emotionally for four years. The synthetic hormone acts to delay puberty rather than halt it completely, and specialists affirm that the effects are reversible, although this remains a controversial topic subject to ongoing research. There are two clear benefits of hormone treatment during puberty: it reduces the psychological distress associated with biological development and it affords a young person and their family time to consider the options that will be available to them later. Ayesha told me that taking the hormone treatment was like pressing pause – her physical body was still predominantly male but with her hormones coshed the effects were much less distressing.

Ayesha attended her psychotherapy sessions wearing heavy make-up and with her eyebrows painted on. The appearance of her eyebrows was incredibly important to her and over time we thought about how they symbolised her sense of identity as well as her emotional state of mind. Some weeks she came late to her appointment because she couldn't get her eyebrows right and was reluctant to leave the house until they were. She watched hours of YouTube tutorials and would painstakingly apply, remove and reapply her make-up. We explored how the appearance of her eyebrows was something within Ayesha's control whereas almost everything else about her physical body was not. In the transference relationship I sensed Ayesha's envy (at times) and hatred (at others) about my female body. This manifested as comments about my appearance, often my hair or my own eyebrows. She would make comments if she thought I'd had my eyebrows done or not bothered to blow dry my hair that had an undertone of covetous resentment. It was as if she was saying,

> You've got what I should have and you're just taking it for granted!

At first I simply noticed her remarks and contained them. Later, as our relationship developed I acknowledged how difficult it must be for Ayesha to accept the painful reality that her body and features were different to mine.

Around the time I first met Ayesha she had also been referred to the adult gender identity service. She was prescribed oestrogen treatment, a more active type of hormone therapy than the synthetic hormone blockers prescribed to delay puberty. These began the process of transforming her body rather than keeping it in limbo. Each week, Ayesha reported on the physiological transformations with delight: decreased facial and body hair and a shrinking of her penis and testes. These changes gave Ayesha the confidence to dress differently. She started wearing skinny fitting jeans and leggings and even talked about creating a fake 'camel's foot' to give the illusion of a vagina. But a vagina was still just that: an illusion. We explored the unbearable truth that Ayesha's body remained predominantly male and that the transformation she longed for was painfully slow and barely perceptible. She talked about wanting breast, bum and hip implants to create a more rounded, feminine body. The images that appealed to her were extreme versions of the female form. She strived to achieve an appearance that seemed (to me) to be cartoonish, like Jessica Rabbit, or unrealistic, like Barbie. As for many young people, not just those grappling with issues of gender identity, Ayesha's influences came from the Internet. Young people are exposed to and have easy access to more varied and more extreme versions of masculinity and femininity than ever before. They are bombarded with images 24/7 dictating how they should look, feel, behave and present themselves sexually.

As the oestrogen therapy began to take effect, Ayesha reported on her tender breasts in a way that was reminiscent of a pubescent girl and displayed curiosity about what further changes to expect. She stopped wearing bras with large cup sizes stuffed with padding and began instead to wear more appropriately fitting underwear. Some of the changes Ayesha reported seemed more couched in fantasy than reality. She talked about having mood swings, 'as if I am on my period' which we both knew could never be the case. I remained respectful but not disingenuous; recognizing that the variations in mood could be associated with adolescence and hormone treatment but acknowledging too that menstruation was something Ayesha would never experience. Over time, I noticed subtle differences in Ayesha's presentation. She began to wear less make-up. Sometimes her eyebrows were barely there. Some weeks she wore casual, loose fitting clothes. It was as if she was growing into becoming a woman rather than creating an extreme and distorted version of one. My work with Ayesha included a fair bit of psychoeducation and a lot of containment. It wasn't my role to condone or condemn her choices, although I did rejoice in her bravery. My role was to be alongside her as she navigated her identity as a young woman in transition, and think with her as she made sense of her experiences. Forming an identity is a process that begins in utero and can last a lifetime, but the bulk of the work happens during childhood and adolescence. Every experience is formative. Every relationship has consequences. Every thought, action and emotion holds significance. Much of what happens from birth to eighteen is beyond children and young people's control – including all of the beginnings, endings and transitions, as well as the ways in which they are managed (or not) by the adults responsible for their care. Our lived and loved experiences provide a mirror to ourselves, our sense of who we are in relation to others and in relation to our self. They shape our identity. They matter. Identity formation is a process that is rarely straightforward or linear. That's why children and young people need adults to listen so that we can help them to make sense of who they are and who they will become.

References

Barnardos, www.barnardos.org.uk/positive-identities-lgbtq-commissioned-work/service-view.htm?id=242895748 (accessed 14 May 2019).
BBC News (2015) http://news.bbc.co.uk/1/hi/health/4530743.stm (accessed 23 April 2019).
Diagnostic and Statistical Manual of Mental Disorders (DSM-V) (2013) American Psychiatric Association.
Freud, S. (1895) *Studies on Hysteria*, Standard Edition Volume II, Hogarth Press, London.
Freud, S. (1930) *Civilization and Its Discontents*, Standard Edition Volume XXI, Hogarth Press, London.
Gender Identity Development Service (2016) Tavistock and Portman NHS Foundation Trust, London.
Hall, G. S. (1904) *Adolescence: Its Psychology and Its Relations to Physiology, Anthropology, Sociology, Sex, Crime, Religion, and Education*, Volume I and II, Appleton, New York.
NHS (2019) www.nhs.uk/conditions/gender-dysphoria/treatment/ (accessed 22 March 2019).
Pirlott, A. G. and Schmitt, D. P. (2014) 'Gendered sexual cultures', In Cohen, A. B. (ed.), *Culture Reexamined: Broadening Our Understanding of Social and Evolutionary Forces*, American Psychological Association, Washington, DC.

Chapter 6

Play

If I ask you to think about play in the twenty-first centur, your mind will probably conjure up images of children and young people alone in their rooms for hours on end, staring at screens and clinging onto hand held devices, as they indulge in online gaming via mobile phones and consoles, such as PlayStation, Xbox and the like. To give an indication of just how popular this type of play has become, type the term 'fortnight' – spelling denotes a period of two weeks – into on online search engine and you are met with the response: 'Did you mean: *fortnite*?' – spelling denotes the popular game launched in 2017 that it seems every child and young person I have met since has become obsessed with. For those that don't know, Fortnite... is an online game deemed suitable for people over the age of twelve due to 'frequent scenes of mild violence' (PEGI, 2017). Apparently it's perfectly acceptable for anyone over twelve to indulge in play that involves frequent mild violence. The most popular versions in the Fortnite series are Battle Royale and Save the World. These are player versus environment, or player versus player games in which gamers compete individually, in pairs or small groups to be the last one standing. They collect resources, build shelters and fight off zombie-type creatures. It's an age-old clash of good versus evil in a battle of survival that has timeless appeal. The visuals in Fortnite are cartoon-like rather than graphic and the game even got people dancing, well flossing, so most parents and carers remained unflustered by it. But it's worth bearing in mind that, because this is an online game with a chat function, and players come in a range of ages and demographics, your twelve (or under)-year-old could be communicating with an adult, anywhere in the world, who could be saying absolutely anything in their ear. Note to parents and carers: the chat function can be switched off.

Many of the console games that grab the attention of the media are licensed as suitable for over-eighteens, the Grand Theft Auto (GTA) and Call of Duty franchises being the most commercially successful and enduring. These games are certified as suitable for adults only because they contain extreme violence, multiple motiveless killings and strong language. They also contain vulgarity and sex, which is why they make the headlines. GTA is billed as an action-adventure game that was first launched in 1997 and has shifted more than 220 million units making it the fifth-highest selling video game franchise of all time. It's a third-person observer game with sex and violence at the fore. In other words, it's voyeuristic. In the original GTA (1997) players witness crime, corruption, street gangs and organised murder, including the killing of police officers. In GTA III (2001) the violence is ramped up and players get to observe sexually explicit scenes, with realistic sound effects and graphics. In GTA IV (2008) players can select from the services of prostitutes, including masturbation, fellatio, and full sexual intercourse, and they also get to choose whether to pay the girls, once their services have been received, or kill them. Many of the (predominantly) boys I've met who access these games are still in junior school and spend several hours a day playing them behind closed doors, often with their parent's or carer's knowledge.

Call of Duty is a first-person shooter game – the player does the shooting – launched in 2003, that has sold more than 250 million units. Injury and death are portrayed in graphic detail. Knives and bullets controlled by the player cut through realistic flesh, splattering realistic blood across the screen. Engaging in these games remains the primary pursuit of many primary school aged children, either with or despite parental permission. Justification for Call of Duty reminds us that players have the option to turn down the blood and turn off the profanity to suit their needs. What exactly are the blood and profanity 'needs' of a prepubescent child?

As an aside, the top three best-selling video game franchises of all time do not feature sex or violence at all. Pokemon (age 7+) has sold 295 million units, Sonic the Hedgehog (age 3+) has sold 350 million units, while Mario (age 3+) has sold 577 million units according to TheGamer, the world's leading source for gaming facts and trends (2017). While I remain troubled by the popularity of violent, sexual and sometimes sexually violent 18+ games among under eighteens, what troubles me more is the propensity of many parents, carers and professionals to either vilify gaming, social media and in some cases the world wide web in its entirety on the one hand, or to turn a blind eye on the other. Digital technology is *not* the root of all evil, poor communication and lack of understanding possibly is. So when a child or young person tells me they are playing games such as GTA and Call of Duty I think with them about their motivations. I ask what they enjoy, or don't, what they understand, or don't, and, most importantly perhaps, how playing the games makes them feel. In other words, I try to make sense of their play.

Dylan

Twelve-year-old Dylan was referred to therapy with concerns about social isolation, depression, anxiety, school refusal and enuresis. The referral had been completed by the school's designated safeguarding lead (DSL), who became involved with the family in Dylan's first term of secondary school, due to concerns about low attendance and poor personal hygiene. I offered two initial consultation appointments for Dylan and his mother but on both occasions they did not attend. On the third attempt, I offered to meet with mother, Sharon and the DSL, Charmaine at school. Sharon told us that Dylan's behaviour was beyond her control. He refused to get up in the mornings and said no one could make him go to school. It seemed he was right, as all attempts to date had failed. I wondered why Dylan was struggling to get out of bed and whether he was getting enough rest. I also wondered if he avoided school because of what might happen when he got there or if his refusal to attend was about wanting to stay with some thing or some one at home. I enquired about Dylan's general health, energy levels, exercise and diet in an attempt to explore and rule in or out any underlying physical or mental illness. Sharon told us that the only thing that Dylan was interested in was gaming. She described him as addicted, stating that,

He's on that damn thing from the minute he opens his eyes.

When Sharon told us that Dylan played GTA, I asked if she was aware of the content. She admitted,

I know it's an eighteen, but they all play it at his age don't they?

I commented that some younger people do access the game but that lots don't. It became evident that there were no boundaries about what Dylan played or how long for and that his obsession with gaming had become so intense that he was not prepared to stop for sleep, food, fluid or toilet breaks. I didn't meet Dylan because his primary need was not for psychotherapy. I had no doubt that his withdrawal into violent and sexual online gaming needed to be explored and made sense of but that could come later. In the first instance, Dylan needed boundaries and relationships that would make him feel safe and contained at home. Without these fundamental elements in place, he did not have a safe space from which to explore. His mother agreed to accept support to help her to access the capable parent part of herself that had become lost and to find ways to reconnect with her son.

Playing

Once upon a time families would sit down together to play a board game. That sounds old fashioned perhaps; but Monopoly, in its various forms, remains the best-selling game of all time – and yes, there is a Fortnite edition, a Pokémon edition and a Nintendo edition. Among my therapeutic resources I have a selection of twenty or so board games, including Monopoly and Scrabble in traditional and junior format, as well as Ludo, Cluedo, Pictionary, Snakes and Ladders, Chess, Draughts and Connect 4. I also have other traditional games that are not confined to a board such as Yahtzee, Jenga, Dominoes and packs of cards. These games remain popular with my child and adolescent clients of all ages and most days I will be invited to play at least one. Board games offer enormous therapeutic value. As the psychotherapist Donald Winnicott (2005) said,

> It is in playing and only in playing that the individual child or adult is able to be creative and to use the whole personality, and it is only in being creative that the individual discovers the self.

The entire business of psychotherapy could be described as playing. It is without doubt a process of creativity, and one where, as Winnicott so eloquently put it, the client has the opportunity to discover his or her self as well as, I would add, the opportunity to be discovered by an interested other. Many of the children and young people I meet for psychotherapy lack the capacity to play because they have never been given the opportunity to learn. I would argue that online gaming, on the whole, requires a different set of skills to being playful with another individual in real life (IRL), although I acknowledge that there are exceptions.

Infants who are not played with are denied the experience of internalising a sense of playfulness, which in turn affects their sense of self. I'm talking about play in its widest sense here: playful interactions, playful facial gestures, playful action songs and playful story telling, as well as more traditional play with toys and games. If we observe an ordinary, good enough mother with her baby we will see how she engages in face-to-face play, cooing, making faces and smiling, with the sole intention of delighting her baby and delighting *in* her baby. This type of play teaches the baby how to be in a relationship with another person and how to mutually create shared pleasure and joy (Stern, 1977). As the infant develops, the mother introduces peek-a-boo type games where she hides and then reveals her face, later she might reveal, hide and reveal again a favourite toy. Again, the main purpose of the play is to have fun, but in this simplest of games, the infant is learning to focus its attention, to bear feeling frustrated when the face/toy disappears and to experience delight when it reappears. Psychodynamic literature, in particular, emphasises the importance of play in early infant-caregiver interactions, yet for many infants and children, their earliest experiences of 'play' have been provided by a screen. Online games are readily available for babies, infants and children from birth upwards including online peek-a-boo and online hide-and-seek. A screen is no substitute for the human face and adults who sanction this – not just now and again but as a replacement for real, live person-to-person play – have been accused of social and emotional neglect, or what has been termed

Urban neglect through technology (Jennings, 2011).

A screen cannot detect the nuances of a baby's reactions and adjust its own responses accordingly. A screen cannot teach a child what it means to be in a relationship, to elicit delight, or to share pleasure and joy with another person. There are a number of reasons why parents and carers might substitute face-to-face play with a screen: laziness, deprivation, neglect, mental ill health or a lack of capacity to play him or herself, but this isn't about apportioning blame. Whatever the reason an infant has been deprived of the experience to play, the effects will always be detrimental and extensive.

The lack of a capacity to play manifests in the psychotherapy room in a multitude of ways. Children might lack curiosity about their own life story, other people, the wider world, the therapeutic space or process or about me. I am endlessly curious, especially when I meet a child or young person for the first time. I might wonder aloud about something I've been told has happened, or hasn't happened, and be curious about what it might mean for them. Sometimes my curiosity is met with a response such as 'it just is' or 'I don't know why' or 'I don't care'. This lack of curiosity demonstrates a lack of playfulness and often illustrates a deficit in the child's experience of play. Other young people display a lack of imagination and playfulness when they are offered the opportunity to engage with art resources in the room. They might respond with, 'what shall I draw?' or 'I can't draw' or 'give me something to copy', and the same can happen when musical instruments are offered and I suggest the young person 'just plays' but they feel unable or unwilling to try. It is worth noting that the lack of capacity for play may be due to developmental delay or disorder. That is not the scope or remit of this chapter and it can be assumed that the children and young people described here do not fit such a diagnosis.

Daphne

Contrary to common misconceptions, the experience of emotional deprivation and incapacity to play is not restricted to families in financial poverty. Ten-year-old Daphne was an only child who presented as precocious and pseudo-adult. Her parents emphasised academic achievement and prized social status above all else. They themselves were high-achievers and high-earners. At the time of the referral, Daphne was studying for exams to determine whether she would be accepted at grammar school and had, not uncommonly, become anxious and overwhelmed. Her parents told me, via telephone consultation, that they were concerned she would,

> buckle under the pressure.

Daphne had lost her appetite and was sometimes refusing meals altogether. I didn't meet Daphne's parents face-to-face because they worked long hours and so Daphne was always brought to her sessions by an au pair. As an infant and younger child, much of the role of parenting had fallen to nannies and professional tutors. There was no questioning the fact that Daphne was bright, but when I met her I was struck by the realisation that she seemed to lack the capacity to play. During our first session I introduced Daphne to the resources in the room. She told me that she had won awards for her art and music and that she had private tuition in painting and piano. She didn't want to engage with the art materials or the musical instruments and I hypothesised that to do so would feel more like work than play. I showed Daphne the board games and she told me that she was a junior chess champion. Surprisingly then, she opted to play Frustration for the duration of the session and throughout every session for the initial six weeks of therapy. The game of Frustration is more about luck than skill. It involves pressing down on a clear dome to shake the dice that determines the number of spaces you can move your coloured pieces around the board. Each player has four pieces that are set on their journey with the shake of a six and each one has to circumnavigate the board once to arrive at the designated safe space marked 'home'. The frustrating part of the game is that if your opponent lands on a space containing one of your pieces, it has to return to the start and you must wait to shake a six before you can begin again. It can be incredibly tedious. Daphne didn't engage with me much during the game. She pressed the dome, said out loud the number on the dice, and counted the spaces as her piece moved around the board – Five - one - two three - frour - five - then she sat back in her chair and waited for me to take my turn. If Daphne landed on one of my pieces and had to send me back to the start there were no signs of pleasure or remorse. If I sent one of her pieces back to the start there were no glimpses of annoyance or frustration. It didn't seem to matter to Daphne who won or who lost, she merely played the game according to the rules. We played Frustration for six therapeutic hours and while it was frustrating, it was certainly not playful.

Following the sixth session I arranged a review appointment with Daphne's parents via video call. They told me that their daughter was much calmer, less anxious and that her appetite had improved. Daphne's mother commented that,

> Talking to you is really helping her

and she requested a further block of six sessions. I was amazed. I wondered what Daphne could possibly be getting from the sessions that, to me, felt monotonous, relentless and mind-numbingly dull. When Daphne arrived for her next session she took Frustration out of the cupboard. I made a clumsy comment,

> Still Frustration,

and realised immediately that my own frustration had influenced my tone of voice. Daphne made eye contact with me for a few

seconds then returned to setting up the game. As we played I noticed her glancing at me between turns. I smiled and continued with
the game. I also realised that Daphne wasn't counting aloud anymore; she was just playing, but she was also observing me, which
marked an important shift. I landed on her piece and she said,

> That's frustrating

and smiled. I agreed and smiled back. Daphne's playful remark
symbolised that she had connected with me in a playful way. The
weeks of simply being with Daphne and playing out the routine of
the simple, repetitive game had provided a container. This was akin
to the turn-taking games of peek-a-boo or hide-and-seek enjoyed
by good enough parents and their young infants. The safe, consistent space had enabled Daphne to learn how to be in a relationship
with me so that we could finally begin to play and create shared
pleasure, something she hadn't learnt how to do before.

It's interesting the things children and young people choose
to share with their parents about therapy. Daphne told hers that
talking to me was helping her to feel better. She *wasn't* talking to
me, but at some level, that we were working out how to make sense
of, she *was* communicating. Perhaps if she'd told her high-flying,
high-achieving, high-expectations parents the truth,

> I go to my therapy sessions and we play Frustration

they would have been less able to see the value of therapy and less
willing to support her to continue to attend.

Samuel

Another young person I worked with, Samuel, *did* use his sessions
to talk with me. He talked about what it was like to be gay and how
he would ever be able to share that with his dad. We talked a lot –
about Samuel's feelings for a boy at college, about his dalliances
with Internet dating and about what it meant for him to be gay in a
family of staunch right wing, highly prejudiced and overtly homophobic men. When I met Samuel's father for the six-weekly review
he said,

> I'm not sure why I'm paying out for him to come here every
> week just to play with Lego.

I don't even have any Lego! But I understand why Samuel had told his father that he came to therapy and played because in a way he did. He played with ideas and hypotheses and fears and fancies, and he played with different ways of building himself and his identity, not using Lego but using thoughts and words and ideas as tiny building blocks instead. Samuel hadn't been ready to share any of that with his dad and his dad hadn't been ready to hear it either. As ever, therapy offered an opportunity to play and Samuel's 'fantasy' provided a vehicle for the truth.

Courtney

Courtney, a girl of eight, could barely read or write. She was struggling to access education, had difficulty forming peer relationships, and was described to me as 'vacant'. Courtney had been terribly neglected and it was suspected from her presentation that she had also been physically and possibly sexually abused. When I met her she could not or would not make eye contact and her impaired speech meant she had difficulty expressing herself verbally. She appeared disconnected from the people around her, the world and her own emotions. During the first therapy session, Courtney sat very still on the couch as her eyes moved around the room, taking in her unfamiliar surroundings. I invited her to explore but she didn't move. I wondered if anything in particular had caught her eye and she pointed to a game of Solitaire. Solitaire is a single player game comprising of a round board with thirty-two coloured pegs lined up in thirty-two holes with a spare hole in the centre. The aim of the game is to remove as many pegs as possible by jumping over one peg with another into an empty adjacent hole. I explained the rules to Courtney and she grasped it immediately. Courtney played Solitaire for the duration of the first session and for the most part of every consecutive session for many weeks. As soon as she realised she had run out of moves she replaced all the pegs and started again, almost without missing a beat.

Courtney had spent time in foster placements, mostly for a week or two at a time, before being returned home to live with her mother, who'd had a number of partners, some of who were alleged to have been abusive towards Courtney. I wondered about the symbolism of the play I witnessed and what it could be communicating about her internal world. I began to gently and carefully voice my observations, saying things like,

It seems as if you've run out of moves

and

I can see you are getting ready to start again.

These were observations about Courtney's observable play, of course, but I was also mindful that they were potentially interpretations about what Courtney was communicating about her history of going in and out of foster care and her repeated experiences of having to start over. As the weeks went on, Courtney seemed to stumble over the pieces. Her handling of the pegs became clumsy and sometimes it seemed as if she was really forcing them into the holes. Again I commented on the observable play,

It seems as if that green peg is struggling to fit into that hole today

and I also wondered to myself about what had been forced where in the past; Courtney into different foster homes where she might feel as if she did or didn't fit, or, perhaps, things being forced into Courtney if the suspicions about sexual abuse were correct. Courtney's solitary game of Solitaire filled much of her early psychotherapy sessions. Over time, the nuances of the play changed gradually as did the duration of time she spent playing the game. By about week eight, Courtney started each session with one game of Solitaire and then moved on to other activities, sometimes other board games or sometimes drawing. Solitaire became a sort of beginning ritual to the sessions and again I pondered about other rituals she might have experienced in the past: the ritual of ending and starting new placements, the introductions and goodbyes, as well as the sometimes ritualistic nature of abuse.

Psychotherapy provided Courtney with a different kind of experience of ritual, one that she could motivate and control for herself. Although her sessions were mostly non-verbal, the opportunity to play allowed Courtney to work something through and make sense of her internal world, at a non-verbal and probably unconscious level. At the three-month therapy review, those adults responsible for Courtney's care reported that she was much calmer at home and more settled in school. She was accessing learning support and

starting to make academic progress and she was playing collaboratively with same aged peers. Courtney had learnt how to play!

Enrique

Enrique invited me to play Junior Monopoly. The game is based
on the original and marketed in a child-friendly way at children
age five to eight years. Fairground rides take the place of London
streets and ticket booths are purchased instead of properties. The
game has low stakes. Players earn two pounds pocket money for
passing GO and pay between one and five pounds to ride the attrac-
tions. Enrique and I spent eight weeks playing Junior Monopoly,
with very little verbal exchange. The sessions often felt boring and
monotonous, sometimes mind-numbingly so. What is perhaps most
striking is that Enrique was an articulate, intellectually capable,
sixteen-year-old. He had been referred to therapy because of his
risk-taking behaviours around drugs and alcohol, which appeared
to be a response to a traumatic family history.

I think that during the early weeks of therapy, Enrique's
mind-numbing play illustrated a desire to numb his mind as a
form of escape, which was also the motivation for his substance
abuse. I also think he wanted to numb my mind, perhaps not consciously, so that I wouldn't be able to think about him or with
him or encourage him to think about his unthinkable past. But of
course I did think. I thought about what was happening between
us, in the transference relationship, and I thought about Enrique's
need to remain detached and defended, which I respected. As well
as representing an escape from the here-and-now, Enrique's play
also suggested a need to re-enact something about his early experiences, of a child aged five to eight. I knew from the referral,
and Enrique knew that I knew, that he had experienced a most
horrific trauma when he was six. His mother, who was due for
release from a lengthy prison sentence for manslaughter at the
time of referral, had stabbed and killed his domestically abusive
father. What an unbearable truth for Enrique to carry with him
and bear. No wonder he sought mind-numbing activities to split
off that part of his internal narrative. Playing a game designed
for a younger child also provided Enrique with the opportunity
to revisit his younger self, the little boy who had been denied the
opportunity to play.

For weeks and weeks we played Junior Monopoly. I absorbed Enrique's projections and felt the feelings he needed me to feel of monotony and mind-numbing boredom. As he began to relax in the space I noticed subtle shifts in the way he related to me that symbolised a developing connection. He made more eye contact and held my gaze for slightly longer. He gave me a fleeting smile when I opened the door to greet him. He nodded in acknowledgement when I commented, 'see you next time' at the end of the session. Enrique needed the experience of playing together *on fair ground* as an antidote to the immense unfairness of his experiences. This provided the foundations for therapy, enabling Enrique to feel safe enough to explore his fears and fantasies. He continued to engage in weekly psychotherapy for two years and we sometimes referred back to the 'fair ground' we created together which, in psychodynamic terms, provided Enrique with a safe base from which to explore.

Times change. Theories, policies and practices evolve. The popularity of different toys, games and consoles comes and goes. But one thing that remains indisputable is that play matters for the healthy emotional, social and psychological development of children. Play is more than a frivolous pastime. As Gibbens (1950) stated, it is nature's way of,

...preparing a child for the serious business of life.

The sessions described in this chapter often felt monotonous and sometimes I wondered what the point of them was. I reflected on their value, in therapeutic as well as monetary terms, just as the parents and carers of the children and young people I supported sometimes did. But those parents and carers also observed calmness where previously there had been chaos, and social isolation was replaced with real-world relationships and connections. Playing together provides a sense of consistency, stability and containment. What these psychotherapy sessions illustrate is that when children and young people are offered the opportunity to play and be playful with a playful and attentive (m)other they develop their capacity for reflection and they begin to make sense of themselves, their worlds and their relationships. This becomes evident both inside the therapy room and in their external worlds.

References

Gibbens, Dr. J. (1950) *Care of Children from One to Five*, Fourth Edition, The Whitefriars Press Ltd., London.

Grand Theft Auto (1997) Rockstar Games, New York.

Grand Theft Auto III (2001) Rockstar Games, New York.

Grand Theft Auto IV (2008) Rockstar Games, New York.

Jennings, S. (2011) *Healthy Attachments and Neuro-Dramatic-Play*, Jessica Kingsley Publishers, London.

Pan-European Game Information (PEGI) (2017) https://pegi.info/page/pegi-organisation (accessed 9 May 2019).

Stern, D. N. (1977) *The First Relationship*, Harvard University Press, London.

TheGamer (2017) www.thegamer.com/top-15-highest-grossing-video-game-franchises-of-all-time/ (accessed 9 May 2019).

Winnicott, D. W. (2005) *Playing and Reality*, p. 73, Psychology Press, London.

Chapter 7

Endings and loss

Generally speaking, there is a split in our collective western cultural consciousness that suggests beginnings are good and endings are bad. We hear of a birth or someone entering a new relationship or being offered a new job and we think of it as a happy time of celebration and send congratulatory greetings. Beginnings are usually a time of hopefulness and anticipation, perhaps coloured with a healthy dose of apprehension. We don't usually embark on a new relationship or start a new job imagining how or when it will end. If we did, we would be thought of as pessimistic or neurotic or even paranoid. Instead, we fantasise about the relationship or the job lasting forever, satisfying us more than our previous relationships and jobs did. When we embark on a new relationship, we can imagine that new person in our life becoming a cherished companion for evermore. New parents feel this way about their babies, however they come into their lives: through biological conception, surrogacy, adoption or some other way. The beginning of a new life is such a cause of celebration that even strangers offer their congratulations! Adolescents in fledgling relationships imagine themselves living together happily ever after. A twelve-year-old boy told me about his 'longest ever girlfriend' and how he could see them getting married and having a family of their own when they were older. They had been a couple for two and a half days and he could not bear to think that his special relationship might one day come to an end.

In contrast to beginnings, when we hear about an ending: of a relationship or job, or the end of a life, we share our condolences and imagine suffering and pain. Often, but not always, things end because they are in some way 'bad'. The job or relationship might not satisfy or gratify us anymore and so we leave it, or are left. As a rule, good relationships don't end and people don't resign from satisfying jobs. People die because they are old or unwell or have been involved in a tragedy: an accident or a murder perhaps, not because they are young and healthy and full of life. We are pitied or consoled because of our losses. Usually, but not always, endings happen for reasons beyond our control, whereas beginnings generally imply more of a choice, even if that is not actually the case. Splitting is a psychological defence. It's one of the ways we try to manage difficult emotions by avoiding them and attaching them to 'other'. Attaching all the negative feelings to endings and putting them in a box marked 'bad' means we can keep beginnings good and untarnished. This is how the split endures.

Therapy beginnings are often preceded by an experience of an ending. As the famous poem states,

The end is where we start from (Eliot, 1941).

For children and young people, in particular, endings are beyond their control and usually happen without their consent. Experiences leading to therapeutic referrals of children and young people regularly include the end of their parent's marriage, the end or imminent end of a loved one's life, the end of a familiar school or home or country of origin. Many young people come to therapy carrying the burden of broken or damaged relationships that have ended. For looked after children, referrers frequently list numerous placement endings, which also, of course, incorporate the end of many significant attachments to birth relatives as well as carers, placement 'siblings', teachers and peers. I once had a first session with an eight-year-old girl in foster care who told me she had experienced eighty-six goodbyes. That was a lot of endings to lug around on her little shoulders.

As a therapist, I try to offer children and young people a different experience of a relationship to the ones they have had before, which have not been experienced as good enough for one reason or another. I offer a different way of relating that models care and compassion, and that is furnished around *their* needs not mine, or their parents' or anyone else's. But it's important to manage their and their families', as well as my own, expectations, and to acknowledge the limitations of therapy, one of which is that it is finite and that our relationship will end. For this reason, every therapeutic intervention should begin with a conversation about when and how it will end. Some therapeutic endings are governed by time-limited or financial constraints that can feel arbitrary. The young person might not have any say in this and they might not feel 'better' when the ending comes. The parent, carer or referrer might not perceive them as 'fixed' and the young person and/ or I might feel less than good enough. Like most feelings, these can be managed and addressed if they are acknowledged and explored. In time-limited work the ending is always in sight and so it makes sense to acknowledge it in the beginning. I might say something like,

> We will meet together for ten sessions and then we will think about how therapy has been for you and then we will say goodbye.

This might sound punitive, but to avoid the reality of the certain ending would be much more painful. I think the reason it can feel difficult for some therapists is because acknowledging the ending at the beginning opens us up to the child or young person's feelings about previous endings and losses that have been shut away in a box. Once let loose, those feelings are likely to become projected onto us. It is our job, of course, to bear the projections, to work with and make sense of them. Some young people are well aware of the box marked 'bad feelings'. One young woman I worked with told me,

> I put all my feelings about my mum's death in a box.

When I asked her about the box she said,

> I threw it away.

Robena

I worked with a seven-year-old girl called Robena. From the beginning, her mother was honest about her own ambivalence towards therapy, which seemed to be about her (mother's) anxiety that Robena would become dependent on it/me. I appreciate honest communication because once fears are named and acknowledged they can be explored and, hopefully, made sense of. Robena's mother, Sureya, appeared to be flagging up something about an insecure attachment; possibly hers, possibly her daughter's, but it was on my radar from the off. Sureya had sought my help because of concerns that her daughter had become sad and isolated. Her mother told me that she wasn't her usual bubbly self and that she had begun to shut herself away, emotionally and physically, from the family. Family comprised of mum, dad, Robena and little brother Joel. When I asked the 'why now' question, I learnt that Sureya's mother was dying. She had been diagnosed with terminal breast cancer six months previously and the care was palliative rather than curative. Robena was emotionally very close to her maternal grandmother and in her early years had been cared for by her when Sureya returned to work. Sureya was honest about her difficulty adapting to motherhood and how she struggled to feel a maternal bond towards baby Robena. This made some sense of the ambivalent attachment style that had been flagged up in the initial consultation. Sureya told me that Robena had,

> Emotionally shut down the minute she found out about her grandma.

I suggested that, as this must be an incredibly difficult time for Sureya, having someone outside of the family to think with about her feelings might help Robena to make some sense of things. Sureya agreed to six sessions of individual psychotherapy for her daughter but cautioned that she,

> Didn't want it go on much longer than that.

The first time I met Robena she talked about her puppy, Pinocchio. She said,

> He's acting funny and doesn't want to play with me anymore.

I wondered what Robena thought about this and she said,

> Maybe he's sad.

I agreed that yes, puppies and people sometimes act differently when they are feeling sad and that idea made sense to me too. She said that Pinocchio had been feeling sad for five months and I repeated aloud, 'five months…' demonstrating that I was wondering about the significance of the time span. I didn't ask any direct questions or make any direct links but I let Robena know that I was listening carefully and trying to make sense of what she was telling me. Robena said she would like to draw a picture of Pinocchio to show me what he used to be like and what he was like now. On one side of the page she drew an animated animal with a big smiley face playing with puppy toys. Overhead she drew a big smiley sunshine and a colourful rainbow and the cage was decorated with colourful flowers. On the other side of the page she drew a down in the mouth puppy under a dark cloud. I said it was very clear to me that things were much sadder now than they were before.

Robena asked what she should draw next and I took the opportunity to suggest we make a calendar together. I told her we would be meeting for six sessions, just the two of us, and then on the seventh week we would be joined by her mum so that we could think about how it had been coming here and that is when we would probably say goodbye to each other. Robena said that saying goodbye would make her feel sad.

During the six sessions, Robena didn't talk very much about her family experiences, but she communicated her feelings about them very clearly indeed. She drew pictures and played out scenarios with animal figures that showed constellations of mothers and daughters and grandmothers and granddaughters. She talked about how things were 'before' and how things were 'now' and told me that the animals felt sad. When one of the old giraffes died, Robena and I made a funeral. She wrapped the animal in a picture she had drawn and made a little box to put it in. She told me that the other giraffes were crying because they wouldn't see the old giraffe again and they had known it for their whole lives. I acknowledged the sadness and the tears about saying goodbye to the much-loved giraffe. I joined in with the funeral ritual. I made explicit the fact that the younger giraffes would never see the older giraffe again but that they would remember her in their minds and still love her in their hearts. Prompted by these words, Robena made a colourful picture. In the centre she drew a gravestone and all around the page she drew hearts and sunshines, flowers and butterflies. When it was finished she told me it was a goodbye picture for her grandmother to take with her to heaven.

Prior to the ending review, Sureya telephoned me to say that her mother had 'passed away' and that the family were making plans for the funeral. She hadn't told Robena because she didn't know what to say. I suggested that she be honest with her daughter and that we could think about it together when we meet, if Sureya could bear it. Sureya shared the news with Robena of her grandmother's death on the way to their appointment with me. When I wondered how Robena felt, she said she felt very sad but also happy because she had been able to say goodbye. She also asked me for the goodbye picture which Sureya agreed to place in the casket. Robena had been helped to work through her feelings, prepare for and make sense of her grandmother's death in a way that felt contained, manageable and good enough. We were also able to say goodbye to each other, acknowledging that the time we had spent together had been a special time and one that we would continue to think about each other in our minds. Robena said,

> But I know you're not going to die and I might need to talk to you again one day if I'm feeling sad.

She also said that we didn't need to have a funeral but that her grandmother would have one and that she would like to go. Sureya was able to bear her daughter's feelings and fulfil her wish to take part in the ending ritual of the funeral. The work with Robena demonstrates beautifully the child's capacity to process endings with the support of a containing and mindful other.

Leon

On the contrary, eight-year-old Leon had been denied the opportunity to know why his grandfather had died or to attend the funeral. They'd had a close relationship before Leon went into care and became estranged from his paternal family. Professionals had delivered the news to Leon about his grandfather's death via telephone but given no explanation. They had also decided that it would 'not be appropriate' for him to attend the funeral due to his age and the circumstances of his grandfather's death. Leon's feelings were unprocessed and, unsurprisingly, spilling out in the form of unruly behaviour. At the point of referral he was described as uncontrollable, unmanageable and on the brink of exclusion from his placement. It was when I asked the 'why now' question that I learnt about his grandfather's recent death through an unintentional overdose of recreational drugs and alcohol.

It is difficult for me to understand why seemingly well-meaning adults deny children knowledge that would help them to make sense of their experiences and feelings. Not knowing is an unbearable position and so inevitably, the space taken up with 'unknowns' gets filled up with worry or fantasy. For Leon, these fantasies included,

> My grandfather was a monster – I'm a monster – He didn't really love me – No-one will love me – I'm unlovable.

Subsequently, his negative beliefs manifested as 'acting-out' angry behaviours. For others they can manifest as 'acting-in' behaviours such as isolation and despair. All too often adults seek to punish or pathologise children when what they really need is containment so that they can make sense of their experiences and their feelings. Questions come to my mind about what is unknowable or unthinkable about and by whom. The majority of children and young people are equipped with innate curiosity and a desire to question everything. If their curiosity is contained, managed and made sense of, those children learn about the world and develop thoughts and feelings about it and themselves. If their curiosity is quelled and their questions remain unanswered or ignored, they learn to stop asking and to split off their feelings. I have engaged in many 'facts of life' conversations in therapy sessions to do with sex, drugs, abortion, suicide, crime and punishment. I know some therapists think that these topics are off limits but I would argue not. Therapy provides a safe space where children and young people can bring their fears and fantasies to be thought about and made sense of – *whatever* those fears and fantasies pertain to. I have explored death with four-year-olds, explained the characteristics of mental illness to a ten-year-old and discussed drugs with eight-year-old Leon. And I have done so confidently and candidly. Leon knew that his grandfather abused substances because he had grown up in that environment. He also knew that it was unlikely that his grandfather, who was a man in his late 40s, would have suddenly dropped dead. So, we talked about drugs – Leon knew that names of several: cocaine, heroin, weed, pills – and we talked about the damage they do to the body. We also talked about how, in some cases, if taken in excess and for a long time, drugs can kill. We thought about the reasons why people might choose to take drugs, given that everyone knows how dangerous they can be. Leon thought it might be because they have nothing else to do, or because they feel angry or sad. In my experience, children are never too young, whatever their age, to be treated with respect and protected from ignorance. They can manage information about all kinds of things if a capacity to manage it is modelled for them. Leon told me that he felt sad about his granddad's death and upset that he hadn't been allowed to attend the funeral. He also said that he was pleased that his granddad wouldn't be sad or angry anymore now that he was dead.

Weaning

In short-term therapy the ending always feels imminent, but in long-term therapy too it's important to acknowledge the ending at the beginning and then, when it's within our sights, to distinguish an ending period that I think of as weaning. With children and young people I tend to offer therapy in blocks. This makes sense to them and their families because it fits with their experience of the academic term. The end of each therapy block gives us an opportunity to pause and reflect, to think back to the reason for referral and the initial hopes and expectations for therapy. I ask questions such as

How are things now? – What's changed? – What still needs to change? – Is this type of therapy still helpful? and Is it time to think about ending?

The review sessions are always collaborative and, wherever possible, include the young person and at least one of their parents or carers. That way, everyone is involved in the process of thinking about ending from the beginning and no one gets a nasty, unexpected surprise when the time comes. In my view, the primary aim of psychotherapy is to be ready to end. It is my job to always hold the end in mind and to be always reviewing the therapeutic goals. My work is non-directive; I don't set the agenda for getting to the end, but I do always hold it in mind. I have come to perceive helping children, young people and their families to manage endings as one of my most important therapeutic occupations.

In long-term therapy, there will naturally be breaks, for the client's or my own family holidays, for public holidays and sometimes for illness. These act as mini endings or practice endings, and as with actual endings, wherever possible they are planned and prepared for together. I say things like,

We have three more sessions and then we will break for two weeks for Christmas,

and then,

We have two more sessions and then we will break for two weeks for Christmas.

With cognitively or chronologically younger children I encourage them to make a calendar to illustrate the number of sessions and the breaks, perhaps writing down the dates but often using images or drawings of their choice. This provides a visual reminder of the sessions and breaks between them, but it also has symbolic value in that we have co-created the structure and the rhythm of therapy together, so that the child can experience a sense of ownership.

Clients and counsellors become attached, which is what facilitates therapeutic work, and so they need time to separate. This can mirror the period of weaning for mother and baby, and also the period of adolescence where the young person learns to separate from their family as they transition to adulthood and independence. Ideally, endings are jointly negotiated, based on a combination of clinical judgement and client wellbeing. They should be thought about as a process rather than a distinct event, a process that starts at the very beginning. The aim of therapy is to be ready and able to end, just as the aim of caring for a baby is to prepare them for adult independence. If earlier separations have been experienced as problematic or traumatic, so too, the emotions provoked by therapeutic breaks and endings can seem to mirror those events. During the initial consultation I will have heard about the baby's first separation, that from the womb, and wondered about how that event was experienced. Was mother conscious or heavily sedated? Did mother and baby stay together or were they separated because one or the other needed special care? If the child or young person is an adoptee I am curious about the separation from their birth family too. Sometimes that is a narrative I have with the parents separately from the child or young person because those stories can be incredibly traumatic. I explore with the family their experiences of other separations too such as mother returning to work, infant starting school, and any other planned or unplanned separations within the family. In my work with looked after children I explore the experiences of separation from birth family and, frequently, separations from multiple placements and carers. Every experience of separation becomes incorporated in a young person's model of ending.

Luca

I seem to have a disproportionate number of referrals of young adolescents in academic Year 7. My hypothesis is that the transition from the (usually) relatively small, nurturing atmosphere of primary school to the larger, more rigorous environment of secondary education evokes feelings from previous transitions that have incorporated separations and endings. Twelve-year-old Luca was a typical example of one such referral. He was a looked after child in residential care who was half a term into his secondary education when I met him. Luca had been in his residential placement for twelve months and had settled well to the routine and the boundaries. My hypothesis was that he experienced containment, probably for the first time in his life. Luca's early years had been neglectful. His mother was addicted to substances and prioritised her own needs over those of her son. The flat where they lived was described as squalid and it was frequented by a series of mother's male friends, boyfriends and dealers. Luca had periods in and out of foster care staying in emergency placements that were always unannounced as a result of his mother's relapses. Children who have been neglected are used to a lack of attention from their parents or carers and situations get set up unconsciously that replicate this so that they experience 'double-deprivation' (Henry, 1974). Their presentation and behaviour often makes them difficult to endear to, meaning that they continue to be overlooked, ignored and neglected. Foster carers offering emergency placements of one or two nights provided Luca with little more than bed, breakfast and an evening meal. There was no time to form a relationship or to offer him a different kind of mothering. Eventually, social care decided to move Luca into longer-term foster care so that he could experience a period of 'consistency'. However, Luca was unable to settle and six separate foster placements broke down. It was then that he was moved into a residential placement. So by the age of eleven, Luca had lived with eleven different families, and experienced dozens of sudden, unannounced endings.

Sadly, stories like Luca's are not unfamiliar in my work with looked after children. There seems to be a prevailing belief, in the general population as well as in the system, that foster care is second best to family care, while residential care is a last resort. I disagree. I have seen scores of children and young people thrive in a residential setting. As with any relationship, the important thing is to find the right match. Often, for children such as Luca who have had a traumatic and uncontaining experience of family life, further experiences within a family provoke them to recreate the trauma and to present as both uncontained and uncontainable. I frequently hear stories from exasperated foster carers and social workers about children who are provided with 'everything they could need' only to smash it to pieces. I hear too about the days out and holidays that the children could previously 'only ever have dreamed of' which they are said to 'go out of their way to intentionally spoil'. These children have had their lives 'smashed to pieces' by well-intentioned – though not always well enough informed – professionals who claim to know what's best for them. I describe professionals this way because, in my experience, information about the history of a child or young person in care is often withheld, diluted, mislaid or lost. My experiences are shared by others who offer therapeutic interventions to looked after children. As Canham (1998) writes,

> I suspect that difficult details about children are withheld consciously or unconsciously for fear that people would not take these children on if they really knew what they had been through and could be like.

For many children like Luca, it's not so much 'better the devil you know' but rather 'this is the only devil I *can* know and this is the only way I know how to survive'. Left unprocessed and unthought about, past experiences remain unresolved and continue to impact on the present in ways that make little sense to the children themselves, or to their carers (Canham, 1999). Subsequent homes and replacement families get smashed, trashed and spoiled. Without the emotional experiences being digested and made sense of, no one can be supported to thrive.

Luca, as I said, had become settled in a residential placement. I think that there are a number of reasons why this kind of 'family' met his needs. Firstly, the relationships available to him were less intimate and therefore less intense than those within a more traditional family home. Staff in residential settings work in shifts. They come and then they go home to their own families or they leave – there tends to be a high staff turnover in residential care. In this way, they are better able to survive – or flee from – the powerful projections foisted on them than a single carer or parental couple with nowhere to go is able to do. They also, the ones that are good enough, tend to have firm boundaries. Rules are rules. They are set in stone, or at least in the company's staff handbook, and they are adhered to vehemently. So often in families, rules about things like Internet or mobile phone use or curfews get bent or broken. This isn't necessarily 'bad' per se; pushing and renegotiating boundaries is a healthy part of ordinary adolescent development. But for children like Luca, who have grown up in boundariless homes, this can feel confusing and uncontaining. In a residential setting there is no negotiation; the boundaries get pushed, of course they do, but they don't budge. It's (mostly) like that in therapy too.

Luca was a willing weekly attendee to therapy who presented as compliant. He arrived on time, remained in the room and left at the designated time. At school, on the other hand, I heard that he wouldn't sit still at his desk, absconded between lessons, left the school premises at lunchtime and sometimes didn't return in the afternoons. For me, the communication was loud and clear,

I'm presenting as uncontained because that's how I'm feeling right now.

What Luca needed was reassurance that the school could keep him safe – he *knew* it cognitively, but he didn't *feel* it emotionally. Luca needed time and support to enable him to trust these new adults in his life, who were many and unfamiliar and who, it was likely, put him in touch with the feelings of living with the many and unfamiliar carers who had been appointed to provide him with care throughout his life. Luca's own sense of internal containment seemed fragile; in other words, he didn't have it in him to feel contained in and of himself. That was the work of therapy; to help Luca to develop a more robust sense of self so that separations, endings and transitions could be more easily navigated without provoking unbearable feelings of falling apart.

Of all the resources on offer in the room, Luca chose to draw. We sat side by side at the table and I observed as he sketched detailed pencil images of cartoon figures, narrating their characteristics and life stories as he drew. He was easy to be with and I was interested in his artistic creations. At first, Luca instructed me to draw too, which I did. I think this was his way of diverting my gaze away from him, which would have been experienced as too intense. I'm no artist, but I tried to draw images that were similar in style to Luca's so that I followed his agenda and my usual style of non-directive working. It is also interesting to note that he positioned himself at my side rather than opposite me, again removing himself from my direct gaze. I always invite the child or young person I am working with to decide where we sit, as well as whether I join in with the activity. In his choices, Luca communicated that he was not yet ready to be looked at. I hypothesised that his early experiences lacked the experience of a holding 'maternal gaze' (Winnicott, 2005). From what I'd read in the referral notes, Luca's substance-addicted mother had been far from preoccupied with her baby. He was therefore denied the experience of being part of a mother/baby dyad, taking mutual pleasure in looking and seeing and delighting in each other. Such experiences are crucial to the development of a sense of self and provide a model for future relationships. Being attended to also helps the infant to develop attention, to bear feeling frustrated and to experience delight (Stern, 1977). Luca's experience of neglectful mothering, on the other hand, will have instilled in him an internal sense of chaos, uncontainment and a fear of falling apart. My sense was that these powerful feelings had been reawakened by his recent transition from a place he experienced as nurturing and holding, to one that felt uncontaining and unfamiliar.

Over the months of Luca's therapy, he continued to draw pages and pages of cartoon characters. I observed subtle shifts in his presentation and use of the space and of me. Luca sometimes added colour to his pencil sketches, usually highlighting a key feature such as a hat or a skateboard. He began to look up from his drawings and make eye contact with me when we spoke, which we did more frequently and more freely. He no longer instructed me to draw too, so that my role shifted to that of observer. When it felt comfortable enough to do so, I shared my observations,

> I'm noticing that character has a bigger head than the others... or I'm wondering if that one is running... or that one with the blue hat reminds me of a character you drew last time...

My comments were intended to let Luca know that I was attending to him and was preoccupied with him, for the duration of his session and also that I held him in mind between sessions. Luca's experience of being held and contained in therapy enabled him to develop an internal sense of containment. He began to settle at school. He made friends as well as academic progress. He was more focused and attentive, and developed a range of interests. Luca and I worked together until the end of Year 7, which turned out to be about nine months. We set our end date around Easter for mid-July, giving a long enough period of weaning for us both to get used to and process the separation. We talked about what it would feel like for Luca to not come to therapy anymore. He said he would be 'a bit sad' at not seeing me, but that he thought he would be ok. I agreed it would feel sad for us to say goodbye, but that I thought he would be ok too. During our final session together, Luca gave me a picture he had made outside of therapy, of coloured-in cartoon figures that shared more than a passing resemblance to him and me, sitting together side by side on a wall *looking* at each other. In red graffiti-style letters Luca had written the words, 'thank you' on the brickwork. I think he was saying thank you for being alongside me and thank you for looking.

Billy

In non-directive therapy, the young person decides what happens within each and every session. Sometimes they come with an agenda of what they do and do not want to talk about, but mostly, the content develops organically as part of the therapeutic process. Much of this, of course, happens unconsciously. It is also important that the young person decides how they would like to say goodbye and mark our final session together. In the lead up to ending, I wonder about this and invite the child or young person to share their ideas, which we think about together. Billy suggested that we take a helicopter ride together for his final therapy session! While that was (regrettably) not feasible, his suggestion did provoke a fruitful discussion about how it would be for the two of us to be flying over the town together, observing what was happening in the houses below. Billy had been referred to therapy because he was experiencing extreme night terrors that were affecting his sleep. He was increasingly anxious when separated from his mother and was starting to refuse school. Billy's early life had been dominated by domestic violence. His mother needed lots of medical attention during her pregnancy due to the impact of physical abuse and when Billy was born, he and his mother spent several months in a refuge. The idea of taking a helicopter ride felt hugely symbolic. Indeed, eight-year-old Billy declared,

> It feels like we *have* been in a helicopter together, looking at the tiny people below us and thinking about what's going on in their houses.

Billy was communicating something about the sense of containment he had experienced in therapy, and the distance it had given him to examine his life from another perspective, enabling him to look at 'the tiny people' and think about what happens 'in their houses' behind closed doors. Billy and I spent his final therapy session making and flying paper aeroplanes. Not quite the same as a helicopter ride, but an appropriation of his idea of us flying together and freeing us up to play. Playing with paper planes also facilitated us to get used to saying goodbye as we launched each one with the words, 'goodbye paper plane' and 'goodbye everyone on board' and to acknowledge the 'going away' part of our ending before we finally said 'goodbye Billy' and 'goodbye Jeanine'.

Rituals

I am in favour of rituals and encourage children and young people to acknowledge their last session both as something special and as something different. It would be all too easy to carry on regardless until the final moments, colluding with the fantasy that we will see each other again, which usually we won't. Some young people try their utmost to avoid thinking about the end and refuse to acknowledge their feelings about it. It is important not to collude. If a young person is struggling to acknowledge their feelings about ending therapy I might think aloud about their other endings that I know about. I might say something particular to the young person in the room, such as,

> It seems difficult for you to think about us saying goodbye... perhaps it feels a bit like when you had to say goodbye to your dad.

Or if I sense that would be too painful or too direct I might say something more generic, such as,

> Most people find endings difficult because they bring up a mixture of feelings and my guess is that you have a mixture of feelings today too.

I'm not telling the young person how they feel – 'you probably feel sad' – but I am letting them know that I have acknowledged that they are feeling *something* even though they are unable or unwilling to name it.

Archie

Some children and young people spend weeks planning their therapy ending, providing us with ample opportunities to wonder about how we might feel about saying goodbye, as well as what we might do to ritualise our ending. Ten-year-old Archie decided that we should have a party and I was happy to oblige. I wondered with him about what we might need and he set about making an ever-increasing list over a period of six weeks: chocolate cake, cheese and onion crisps, ham sandwiches, blackcurrant squash, loud music and presents. I could see no good reason to refuse and told Archie that I thought a party was an excellent idea. When I had first met him twelve months previously, he had told me in no uncertain terms that he thought therapists were nosey busybodies, and that therapy was pointless. Over the year, he engaged tentatively at first and then more fully in thinking about his experiences of domestic abuse. With Archie's permission, I shared our plan for a party with his mother and she suggested that she would help him to make a cake that he could bring to the final session. I agreed to supply the other snacks and suggested that we make something together in the session that we could exchange as gifts. Archie agreed. I thought this would avoid any awkwardness about buying an appropriate and affordable gift and would also give us something to work on together in the final session. The planning, thinking and preparation was a collaborative process and I thought with Archie about the symbolism of a party, both as a way of commemorating the work we had done together in therapy, and as a way of celebrating how much more settled he was than when I first met him. I also acknowledged that our party sounded as if it would be full of food and music and activity and I wondered if there would be space for us to think about the difficult feelings associated with saying goodbye. Archie said there probably wouldn't be space for that. When the day of the party arrived, I laid out a picnic of cheese and onion crisps, ham sandwiches and blackcurrant squash. I fired up my laptop with YouTube at the ready to play loud music. On the table I set out craft materials and I waited. And I waited and I waited and I waited until the realisation dawned on me that Archie wasn't coming. I remained in the room throughout Archie's final session and reflected on the work we had done together. I used the craft materials to make him a card and inside I wrote that it had been a pleasure to work with him, that his ending therapy was a celebration but also that it provoked sadness about saying goodbye.

In my experience, it is not uncommon for children and young people to miss their final session. But because we have worked through the ending as a *process*, rather than a one-session event, we will have already acknowledged and made sense of the feelings that endings can provoke. Archie told me in advance that there 'wouldn't be space' to think about the difficult feelings, and in the end he left them with me to process in his absence. When a child or young person misses their last session, I respect their decision to do so but I don't collude. I stay in the room and I reflect on my own feelings and those that might belong to the child. I write a letter or a card to say goodbye and, if it seems appropriate, I acknowledge that saying goodbye in person would perhaps feel too painful.

Aneska

I worked with Aneska throughout her mid adolescence. She was twelve when we met and almost eighteen when therapy ended. There was a period around her thirteenth birthday when we met twice a week. Aneska was academically bright and a high achiever educationally as well as in music and sport. She strived for perfection in all areas and set herself incredibly ambitious goals. She came to therapy in a state of high anxiety and struggled too with disordered eating, restricting her intake of calories to a sometimes dangerous minimum and occasionally binging and vomiting. Given this profile, Aneska was, not surprisingly, something of a model patient. She arrived on time, left on time, was receptive to my ponderings and interpretations and made good use of the therapeutic space. Throughout the five-year therapeutic intervention, Aneska had not one single absence, other than for planned breaks. We began thinking about the ending at the start of the spring term and set a date that coincided with the school summer break. Throughout those twelve weeks, we reflected together on the Aneska who first came to therapy, the girl who was unwell and underweight with a fragile sense of self, compared with the physically and psychologically healthy young woman who was preparing for university. Aneska made dozens of drawings throughout her therapy that illustrated graphically her internal world and we spent time revisiting them and selecting what she wished to do with them throughout her period of 'weaning'. There were some images that Aneska wanted to keep and others that she chose to destroy, for a variety of reasons that we explored and made sense of. The images created during her most difficult year of therapy were the most painful ones to reflect upon, but doing so allowed Aneska to make sense of her younger self and process the feelings associated with that time. As the date for Aneska's end session approached, I had a sense of her gradual detachment from me and from the therapeutic process. She continued to attend weekly and punctually but I was aware that she felt more distant. On the day of her final session, Aneska sent me a message to say that she was unable to come due to a 'deadline' at school. Because this was so untypical, I couldn't help but wonder about the difficulty Aneska had in facing the 'deadline' – literally, the finish line of therapy and the death of our therapeutic relationship. We rescheduled the session for later in the week and once again Aneska made a late cancellation, this time citing 'feeling unwell'. I offered one further session for us to say goodbye but instead of arriving for her session, Aneska posted a card through my door. In it she thanked me for 'bearing with' her and said that she felt ready to go to university.

Elsie

Sometimes it is the family, rather than the child or young person, who is unable or unwilling to bear the ending. When working with young people, it is important to notice and differentiate between 'did not attend' (DNA) and 'was not brought' (WNB) in relation to all missed sessions. Recording a missed session as DNA implicitly places the onus on the client for non-attendance, whereas often, particularly with younger children and young people, the responsibility lies with the parent or carer and so WNB is a more accurate recording. Elsie's referral to therapy came six months after the death of her father to cancer. The thirteen-year-old and her mother, Jo, sobbed openly throughout the initial assessment, illustrating the rawness of their unprocessed grief. The experience of being in the room with them was excruciating, such was the intensity and the unbearableness of their pain. During that first meeting I heard about multiple other losses. Jo's grandfather died during her pregnancy with Elsie. Jo's mother died a year after the birth of Jo's second child, Aiden, and her father was being cared for in a nursing home following a diagnosis a year ago of dementia. Elsie's paternal grandmother lived in New Zealand with her second husband. Her first husband, Elsie's paternal grandfather, died eight years previously, when Elsie was five. The family had experienced so much death, there was no wonder they were struggling to come to terms with their most recent bereavement. I wondered how they managed their sadness and Jo told me that they often cried together.

Grief is, of course, a deeply personal experience. I was struck by Jo and Elsie's *shared* outpouring of grief and their crying *together*, which seemed to symbolise a spilling out rather than a thinking through of their emotions. I wondered too whether crying together was a way to externalise, and therefore split off, those personal feelings that were perhaps too painful to contain. Elsie's entire life, from pre-birth onwards, had been punctuated by death. I wondered whether her tears were a learned response from an openly demonstrative mother. The therapeutic work with Elsie focused on making sense of her experiences. At first her tears struck me as a way to get rid of rather than acknowledge her feelings in response to loss, which were unprocessed and therefore sore and easily provoked. We used the sessions to explore her beliefs about life and death and life *after* death, both in relation to the deceased and those left to mourn – was it ok to be happy after someone close to you had died? What would it mean if you were? I sometimes introduce resources to the children and young people I work with if I think it might be beneficial. One book that I find particularly helpful in trying to make sense of death is the 'Seeds of hope, bereavement and loss activity book' (Jay, 2015). The book encourages an awareness of nature and the cyclical nature of life. It reminds us that life is part of death, which is a part of life. The activities encourage recollections of happy memories about someone who is loved and lost, reminding us that, just as life and death are interlinked, so too are happiness and sadness. This avoids the temptation to split, to be black or white or either/or, which can be enticing. Elsie and I reflected upon the certainty of death, as well as the uncertainty about where and when and how it will come. She was keen to explore these issues, both at a personal and at a more existential level. She remained sad about her father's death, which was appropriate, but she began to grieve him in a way that allowed her to acknowledge and manage a complexity of feelings, including enjoyment of her life now and happiness in relation to the times she, her brother and her parents had spent together as a family.

After about ten sessions Elsie and I decided together that she felt better able to contain her emotions. Her different feelings made sense to her now and had been named and processed so that they no longer spilled out, nor needed to be split off. I invited Jo to join Elsie and me for a final therapy review and shared that Elsie felt ready to end therapy. We spent the joint session reflecting on the themes and process of therapy and I suggested we arrange a time for Elsie and I to meet for a final ending session. Jo said she didn't have her diary with her and would get in touch. When I hadn't heard from her a week later, I sent an email to give a gentle nudge. Jo replied a few days later but said she couldn't make a date yet as the family had 'lots going on'. Again I waited for a week before I sent another email, reminding Jo that we needed to make a date for a therapeutic ending. She didn't reply. My hypothesis was that, for Jo, the act of making an ending was too unbearable. In some ways, perhaps, that final session would have symbolised the finality of a funeral.

That period of time between death and burial can be experienced as a state of limbo. For many, it provides a tantalising opportunity to deny their loss and create a pretence that the deceased has gone away and will return. A funeral puts an end to the fantasy with a familiar cultural ritual that symbolises the end. Some people choose not to attend the funeral of a loved one for that reason, or they forbid their children from attending to 'protect' them from the finality of death. I think that denial of the truth is never a good idea. Rather than protect, it displaces the feelings or attempts to split them off which is likely to set up difficulties later. I can't know what Jo's motivation was for failing to arrange a therapy ending for her daughter, or Elsie's feelings about being denied the opportunity to say goodbye to me. But, as with Aneska and all the children and young people I work with therapeutically, Elsie and I had worked through the therapy ending as a process. I wrote to her to say goodbye.

The end

Frequently, psychotherapists and counsellors are tempted to leave the door ajar for children and young people to return to therapy some time in the imagined future. I advise caution. Occasionally it might be appropriate to take a break from therapy with the intention to resume at a later date. But I strongly believe that this should be the exception rather than the norm. Considering an ending as an extended break, or indeed treating therapy referrals and discharges like an ever-revolving door, denies the reality of ending and splits off feelings associated with saying goodbye. In order to experience a good enough ending, we need to be clear – in our own minds as well as with the children and young people we support – that that is exactly what it is: the end. I think there is something about endings that people seem set up to avoid. Have you ever watched a television series, a drama perhaps, with its plot line twisting and turning in each episode, building to a finale when we hope to finally get an answer to the question of whodunit or will they/won't they, only for the producers to leave us hanging with the promise of a next series? I think that leaving the therapy door open can be a bit like that. It dodges the ending, denies the opportunity for closure and disavows the complexity of emotions. The case of the unfinished television series amounts to lazy writing. The case of the unfinished therapy signifies negligence. Consider too a relationship that isn't working out. One party might commonly say to the other,

> I think we need a break.

When what they really mean is,

> This relationship has no future, we should split up.

I wonder why people can't they just say that. They might argue that they are being kind, protecting the other person's feelings, rather like the social worker who doesn't let a child in their care attend the funeral of their grandfather, or the mother who doesn't arrange a therapy ending for their daughter. They tell themselves it would be too painful and that it is for the other person's own good. I think they are wrong. I think they are demonstrating denial and inviting collusion with a fantasy, something that, as therapists, we must be aware of and do our best to resist. So when I'm thinking about and planning for a therapeutic ending, I call it an ending. To digress slightly, I also call a death a death. Euphemisms are confusing and deny reality.

A further temptation is the one to keep in touch with a client after the 'final' session. To say goodbye with words such as,

> Let me know how you're getting on

or

> It would be good to hear from you.

Again, this functions to deny the finality of the ending. It also puts pressure on the child or young person to do well and to report back to you that they are. If they or their family want to contact us again they will, they have our details. To say, 'let me know…' or, 'it would be good to hear…' is self-serving; it's about satisfying my need to know rather than the other person's need to tell and that's not how therapy works. Of course I'm curious. Of course I wonder about the hundreds of children and young people I have supported, many of whom are now adults, perhaps with jobs and homes and families of their own, perhaps not. Mostly I will never know. Very occasionally, my path crosses that of a former client. We chat, politely enquire how each other is and then move on with our separate lives.

But then there is social media. Over the last decade I have received dozens of friend requests from the young people I work with, have worked with previously and their families. The implementation of General Data Protection Regulation in 2018 prompted us all to rethink the way we store and share data. It also encouraged me to update my privacy policy to include the following statement,

> I do not accept friend requests from clients, former clients or families on social media.

This clear, unambiguous assertion is published on my website and shared with all families at the point of contracting. It is a further example of considering the end at the beginning and avoids any awkward conversations afterwards. As with any safeguarding or boundary issue, if the subject arises, I can refer the child, young person or family back to the contract and say,

> Look, here it is, the place where we agreed that I would not accept your friend request.

If the matter arises during the therapy, I explain to the child or young person that our relationship remains within the therapeutic boundary of time and place in order to protect our individual privacy as well as that of our friends and families. I have peers who accept ex-clients as friends on social media, reasoning that once the professional contract is terminated, it is a legitimate way of keeping in touch. I do not agree. I think it crosses a boundary and, for me, would feel like inviting the ex-client into my personal life. Clients have fantasies about their therapists and I believe those fantasies should be maintained rather than contaminated by access to each other's social media profiles, even after the therapeutic relationship has ended. Imagine accepting a friend request from an ex-client and finding out that everything they told you about their life during the therapy was untrue. How awful to be left with that feeling and not be able to explore it with the client themselves.

Along with the lure of social media, comes the lure of Google. I fully expect to be googled by parents, carers, social workers, referrers, children and young people, readers, supervisees, trainees, critics and colleagues. It is part and parcel of being alive in the twenty-first century. I have a professional website and a professional Twitter profile which are designed to be read and promote my work as a psychotherapist. I also use other social media for non-professional purposes and these are set up to protect my privacy, as much as possible. I know of professionals who search their client's social media profiles or google their names out of curiosity. For me, technological snooping crosses a boundary and feels intrusive. If I want to know more about a child, young person or family I'm working with, I ask I don't spy. If they are inquisitive about me I encourage them to do the same. Even though I don't share personal details, I think this models honesty and respect and it holds the therapeutic boundary. If a child or young person chooses to google me or search for me on social media, so be it, but I still invite them to share what they find, or can't find and remain curious or cross about, so that we can think about that together in session. How we think about children and young people *after* therapy should be as ethically informed as how we think about them *during* therapy. Any decisions or dilemmas should always be resolved with *their* best interests in mind, not ours, whether those decisions are to do with making an ending, declining a friend request or negotiating what happens afterwards.

An ending is a demarcation between what has come before – a therapeutic intervention, a relationship, a life – and what will come afterwards. As I move towards each and every therapeutic ending I hold in mind that with endings come new beginnings.

References

Canham, H. (1998) 'Growing up in residential care' (p. 55). In Briggs, A. (ed.), (2012) *Waiting to Be Found*, Papers on children in care, Karnac, London.
Canham, H. (1999) 'The development of the concept of time in fostered and adopted children', In Briggs, A. (ed.), (2012) *Waiting to Be Found*, Papers on children in care, Karnac, London.
Eliot, T. S. (1941) 'Little Gidding' from *Four Quartets*, Harcourt, London.
Henry, G. (1974) 'Doubly deprived', In Williams, G. (ed.), (2004) *Internal Landscapes and Foreign Bodies*, Routledge, London.
Jay, C. (2015) *Seeds of Hope Bereavement and Loss Activity Book*, Jessica Kingsley Publishers, London.
Stern, D. N. (1977) *The First Relationship*, Harvard University Press, London.
Winnicott, D. W. (2005) *Playing and Reality*, Psychology Press, London.

Index

For Product Safety Concerns and Information please contact our EU
representative GPSR@taylorandfrancis.com
Taylor & Francis Verlag GmbH, Kaufingerstraße 24, 80331 München, Germany

* 9 7 8 0 3 6 7 1 4 9 4 0 6 *